AVOIDING BREAST CANCER

While Balancing Your Hormones

The FEM Centre Breast Care Program

by Joseph F. McWherter, M.D.

A & Rosebud

Dallas, Texas

Copy Editor: Karen Patterson

Exercise photographs: 76 Images (www.76images.com)

Exercise routines: Joy Cole (www.joysstudio.com)

Breast anatomy and breast self-exam illustrations: Copyright © 2005 Nucleus Medical Art,
    All rights reserved. (www.nucleusinc.com)

Cover photograph: © 2005 JupiterImages Corporation

Back cover photograph: Courtesy of Banks Photography (www.banksphotography.com)

Published by A. E. Rosebud, LLC, PO Box 814662, Dallas, Texas 75381.

First edition. Printed and bound in the United States of America.

ISBN 0-9772487-0-4

This book is dedicated to my wife, Becky.

I could never have completed this project
without your continuous help and support.

I love you!

TABLE OF CONTENTS

List of Illustrations i

Acknowledgements iii

About the Author v

Foreword vii

Preface...ix

Introduction xi

Chapter 1
Cancer and Breast Health 1

Chapter 2
Causes of Breast Cancer 5
    DNA Damage 6
    Cell Matrix Damage...7
    Risk Factors 8

Chapter 3
Estrogen Explained...13
    The Three Types of Internally Produced Estrogens 15
    The Externally Produced Estrogens 20

Chapter 4
Estrogen and the WHI Study..**25**
How Does Estrogen Interact with the Breast Cell? 27
The Three Kinds of Estrogen Metabolites 28
Hormonal Therapy "Window of Opportunity" 32
Summary: Estrogen and the WHI Study 33

Chapter 5
A Woman's Hormonal Transitions **35**
The Reproductive Compartments 35
Before Birth 37
Puberty 39
Life Phases After the Onset of Puberty 42

Chapter 6
The FEM Centre Breast Care Pyramid..**57**

Chapter 7
Exercise, Stress Reduction, and Nutrition **59**
Exercise...59
Daily Breast Massage and Chest Exercise 69
Stress Reduction 71
Nutrition — The FEM Centre Nutrition Plan 74
The Five Dietary Principles to Promote Breast Health.............77

Chapter 8
Detoxification: The C.A.N. Program and Chelation **107**
The Cellular Matrix...109
Food and the Second Brain...111
Liver-Intestinal Detoxification System.......................................114
C.A.N. Program (Cleanse, Add, Nourish)..................................120
Chelation Therapy 124
Additional Therapies..126
Additional Tests 127

Chapter 9
Balancing Hormones..**131**
The Effects of Hormones..133
Estrogen Applications 137
Progesterone 142
Testosterone 148
Pregnenolone 151
DHEA 153
Thyroid Hormones 156
Melatonin 161
Cortisol 164
Insulin...166
Human Growth Hormone 168

Chapter 10
Breast Care Nutrients...**171**
A Four-Component Breast Care Supplement Program 172
Iodine..173
Omega-3 Fatty Acids (Fish Oil)....................................177
Multivitamin Supplement..178
BreastSecure..184
Other Supplements 189

Chapter 11
Mammograms/Thermograms: The Warning Signs and
Early Detection of Breast Cancer **191**
Breast Self-Examination 191
Thermography...194
Screening Mammograms 196
Self-Exam, Thermogram, Mammogram —
    Who and How Often?..199

Chapter 12
Male Wellness: Being a Partner in Health **203**

Chapter 13
Breast Cancer Survivors 209

Epilogue 219

Appendix A
Detoxification Questionnaire 223

Appendix B
The 21-Day Detoxification Diet 225

Appendix C
Daily Regime & Regular Interval Regime
(Plus Things to Avoid) 233

Appendix D
The Glycemic Index 239

Appendix E
Resources 243

Bibliography 245

Glossary 277

Index 301

LIST OF ILLUSTRATIONS

Figure 1.   The cancer-initiation-to-cancer-propagation path 6

Figure 2.   Anatomy of the breast 14

Figure 3.   The effects of 17β-HSD and aromatase on the
            production of estradiol in the breast and fat cell 17

Figure 4.   The different effects that 2-hydroxyestrogen,
            4-hydroxyestrogen, and 16alpha-hydroxyestrogen
            metabolites have on the breast cell 31

Figure 5.   A woman's reproductive compartments 35

Figure 6.   The twenty-eight-day menstrual cycle 40

Figure 7.   A woman's hormonal transitions 42

Figure 8.   The FEM Centre Breast Care Pyramid 57

Figure 9.   The endocrine hormonal pathway 110

Figure 10. The chain of events related to intestinal problems 119

Figure 11. Cholesterol-derived hormone pathways 137

Figure 12. Estrogen/progesterone/testosterone levels
            during life transitions 142

Figure 13. Human growth hormone, DHEA, pregnenolone,
            and melatonin levels during life transitions 154

Figure 14. The effects breast care nutrients have on estrogen 172

Figure 15. Results of iodine loading tests on nine consecutive breast
cancer patients..175

Figure 16. Breast self-exam — left, using a circular motion;
right, using a vertical, up-down motion........................193

ACKNOWLEDGMENTS

I would like to thank my patients, who have been my teachers and provided the clinical knowledge required to write this book.

Karen Patterson, whose editing skills added clarity to this book.

Dr. Clark Ridley, my associate and fellow obstetrician/gynecologist, whose medical experience and knowledge helped fill in the gaps.

The staff of our detoxification program, Toni Bilbrey and Cherie Head, for providing valuable clinical input in the field of nutrition and detoxification.

Special thanks to Joy Cole for consulting on the exercise section and providing our patients with wonderful training regimens.

And the valued members of the FEM Centre and Energy Health Centre staff, including:

Dr. Patrick Mulcahy, Family Practitioner
Gayla Campbell, Nurse Practitioner
Shelagh Moore, Nurse Practitioner
Emily Mueller-Kuentz, Acupuncturist
Linda Judd, Acupuncturist

ABOUT THE AUTHOR

Joseph F. McWherter, M.D.
FACOG, FACS

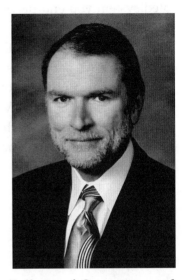

Dr. McWherter received his undergraduate degrees in physics and mathematics in 1973 from the University of Texas at Austin. Upon attending the University of Texas Health Science Center at Dallas, he was awarded a medical degree in 1977 and completed his residency in Obstetrics and Gynecology in 1981. Dr. McWherter is a Fellow of the American College of Obstetricians and Gynecologists, Fellow of the American College of Surgeons, and holds memberships in the American College for Advancement in Medicine, the American Academy of Anti-Aging, and the Endocrine Society. In addition to being a diplomat of the American Board of Chelation Therapy and the Board of Oxidative Medicine, he also has served as chairman of the peer-review planning committee and speaker for the Integrative Medicine for Anti-Aging Conference and Exposition.

Dr. McWherter is Medical Director of the FEM Centre and Energy Health Centre Clinics in Colleyville and Fort Worth, Texas. He has helped thousands of women find optimal health and wellness through hormonal balancing. As an innovator in the fields of women's health and anti-aging, Dr. McWherter's approach to health care addresses the need for an increased awareness of using preventive measures to *avoid* diseases such as breast cancer.

"Traditional medicine views the body as a combination of individual components that function independently of one another. Instead of treating the gastrointestinal system, the cardiovascular system, the immune system, the neurological system, and the hormonal system as separate entities," he says, "I view them as one unified family. Everything in your body is interrelated. If you look at each function as an isolated system you end up treating only the symptoms of a disease, not the root problem."

Dr. McWherter is on the forefront of natural hormonal replacement therapies as well as functional and nutritional medicine. He has developed a unique approach to the health issues facing the contemporary woman. Dr. McWherter's "lifetime wellness" protocol stresses detoxification of the body, balancing the hormones, reinforcing the immune system, and adjusting the diet to provide the body with proper nutrition. His program allows women to experience the life-enhancing benefits of hormonal replacement safely while avoiding their number one fear, breast cancer.

FOREWORD

Avoiding Breast Cancer While Balancing Your Hormones is a much-needed book. Breast cancer is occurring in epidemic proportions, currently affecting one in seven women in the United States.

Conventional medicine has little to offer. Its treatments do nothing to address the causative issues of cancer, and the standard toxic therapies have shown little success in over 30 years of treatment, and billions upon billions of dollars spent.

Dr. McWherter has written an important book that helps the patient find effective ways to avoid breast cancer. In addition, this book gives the reader specific recommendations to help address the underlying cause(s) of developing cancer. This book needs to be read by patient and physician alike.

When there is a diagnosis of cancer, conventional physicians are quick to recommend surgery, chemotherapy and radiation. I don't believe that cancer develops because of a deficiency of surgery, chemotherapy or radiation. Cancer develops from a variety of factors, including exposure to toxic chemicals and synthetic hormones.

Dr. McWherter eloquently writes how these disrupt the cellular matrix, permitting cancer cells to grow and grow. Only by implementing a holistic plan can you reverse this process.

Such a plan can be found in this book. As a practicing holistic physician, I have witnessed the benefits my patients receive from a more natural approach.

The pharmaceutical companies want us to believe that a cure for cancer will be found by a "magic-bullet" drug. This will never occur. Drugs generally block receptors or poison enzymes in the body. I don't believe we were designed to have our receptors blocked or our enzymes poisoned. Through the use of natural items, these receptors and enzymes can be nourished.

The body has a wonderful healing capacity, given the chance. The recommendations in this book can provide the body with the chance to heal.

David Brownstein, M.D.
www.drbrownstein.com
Author: *Overcoming Arthritis*
The Miracle of Natural Hormones
Overcoming Thyroid Disorders
Iodine: Why You Need It, Why You Can't Live Without It
Salt for Your Health

PREFACE

The desire to remain healthy has never seemed so powerful, especially with the surge of baby boomers entering their midlife years. By 2025 it is estimated that an astounding 20 percent of the population will be over 60 years of age. Many of these folks will strive for an energetic, active lifestyle that may include a shift in careers, a cosmetically restored youthful appearance, prevention of chronic diseases, and spiritual satisfaction. In order to achieve these healthy aging goals one must be proactive and begin a wellness program, which includes hormonal balancing.

For the mature woman, the pathway of healthy aging can lead to an entire life of being sexy and full of zest. Unfortunately, almost a quarter of a million of these women will have their journey interrupted by the diagnosis of breast cancer.

The apparent lack of effective preventive measures, along with epidemic numbers of cases, has led to breast cancer becoming a major health concern for most women at midlife and beyond. Yet, millions will suffer from a plethora of other chronic diseases whose treatment costs are part of the staggering 70 percent of our health care dollars spent on an aging population. It should be obvious that the current traditional medical approach is not meeting our needs and therefore must change, as the health care system itself is in danger of collapsing.

The material presented in this book is designed to address this challenge by integrating the best of traditional and complementary medicine into a wellness program that allows you to balance your hormones while avoiding breast cancer. As you will discover, the steps that one takes to protect the breasts also diminish the risk of chronic diseases of aging by improving the overall health of the heart, brain, and bones.

My book focuses on the following topics: 1) examination of the relationship of estrogen to the breast; 2) understanding the conclusions of the WHI study and how they affect you; 3) a review of the physiology of the female reproductive system and exploration of a woman's life transitions in the context of breast health; 4) an explanation of how the FEM Centre Breast Care Program helps you achieve hormonal balance, including the use of estrogen replacement, while avoiding breast cancer; and 5) applications of the program to a breast cancer survivor or a male partner's health.

A discussion of the biochemistry involved in the relationship between hormones and cancer is necessary, but every attempt has been made to simplify the scientific complexity of the subject matter. While some may choose to read the book in its entirety, others can skip to Appendix B and begin the 21-day detox diet along with the daily suggestions listed in Appendix C. Once the detox diet is completed, a chart of suggested foods and supplements along with a meal and exercise log can be printed from the FEM Centre website (femcentre.com/abc_chart.html).

Understanding the topics presented in this book should: 1) expand your wellness knowledge base; 2) help you filter out incorrect or sensationalized claims; and 3) provide answers to commonly asked hormone questions.

In closing, I would like to say this to my current patients: My original intent was for the book to be directed toward helping patients digest the flood of new information presented during an office visit. There is a great deal of material that must be covered during the allotted time. So, to avoid confusion and frustration resulting from information overload, I suggest you go home and read those sections in the book that address what was discussed in the office.

The one ingredient that cannot be supplied by this book is "compliance." Without compliance there can be no long-term prevention. To become proactive in the prevention of breast cancer and to regain vitality, follow the advice in this book, and commit to making a "change for life."

Joseph F. McWherter, M.D.

INTRODUCTION

What I have tried to communicate in this book is that which I have learned from administering to my patients. A very wise physician was quoted as saying: "When all else fails, listen to your patients, for not only will they provide you with a diagnosis but also a treatment plan." And so I began to listen to my patients.

The older I got, the better listener I became. What I heard eventually led me to redefine my entire approach to medicine. Rather than simply treating symptoms as taught to me by my initial traditional medical training, I now began to address causes. Most importantly, prevention became my priority, as opposed to waiting for the onset of disease and then attempting to intervene. Pharmaceutical drugs were no longer the mainstay of my treatment protocols.

To acquaint you with my background, I have been a clinician who has specialized in obstetrics and gynecology for almost 25 years. A clinician is a doctor who provides direct care to patients and understands that medicine is an art based on scientific principles. My initial training was influenced by a traditional medicine curriculum that was concerned mainly with intervention and not prevention of disease.

In addition to practicing gynecology, for many years I was active in the fields of obstetrics and reproductive endocrinology. Having been the medical director of a successful *in vitro* fertilization clinic allowed me to investigate the intricate functions of the female and male endocrine systems, while providing obstetrical care reinforced my appreciation of the physiologic miracle of pregnancy. Part of my continuing role as a gynecologist involves performing pelvic surgery. Visualizing and surgically correcting pathological conditions arising in the female pelvis has underscored the pathway of transition from functional to structural problems.

The sum of these diverse but interrelated experiences has proved to be invaluable in my understanding of the role hormonal changes have in a woman's life transitions.

A major impetus behind my change in direction to preventive health care arose from the fact that my practice matured age-wise as I did, so that the vast majority of women who seek my services are over forty. Their needs differ from those experienced during the child-bearing years. Instead of dealing with pregnancy-related issues, the symptoms now most often verbalized included lack of energy, waking up in the middle of the night and not being able to return to sleep, weight gain about the midsection, a diminished sex drive (which in some cases has resulted in marriage difficulties), anxiety, depression, bowel irregularities, muscle and joint aches, hair loss, hot flashes and night sweats, fuzzy memory, and an overall feeling that things were not as they should be. Many patients have also begun to suffer from what are known as the chronic diseases of aging such as breast, colon, and assorted other cancers; diabetes; arthritis; lupus; hypertension and associated heart ailments; skin disorders that included psoriasis and rosacea; colitis; and chronic fatigue and fibromyalgia. Practicing medicine for over a quarter of a century, I have observed that these diseases seem to be occurring not only with greater frequency but at earlier ages.

My initial approach to resolve these undesirable changes of aging involved the use of a pharmaceutical agent for each individual symptom. Eventually, I found that traditional medicine offered little if any explanation of the underlying causes for these problems and provided little direction regarding their prevention. There was a paucity of information about what triggered the initiation of these chronic diseases, and the only thing one could do was to anticipate their onset and treat the accompanying symptoms.

It was not uncommon to see a woman in midlife be on three or four medications, which included antidepressants, gastric reflux inhibitors (to relieve heartburn), regulators of bowel function (constipation, diarrhea, or both), non-steroidal pain inhibitors (headaches, joint and muscle pain), and sleep aids. Symptoms that I treated would temporarily resolve, or new ones would sprout up out of nowhere.

And still there was no end to the onset of chronic diseases, especially breast cancer. My clinical observations eventually led me to conclude that this was really a Band-Aid approach, which proved to be less than satisfactory over the long term since the underlying health issues were never really addressed.

I then made a commitment to reinvent my medical practice, which started by attending complementary or functional medicine courses. The resulting new concepts were gradually integrated into my practice with amazing results. Women actually started to feel better. Becoming more confident with these protocols allowed me to begin to develop my own, which were specifically tailored to those issues experienced by women at midlife and beyond.

Treating thousands of patients has led me to the initial conclusions that three basic systems must be addressed in order to cause a decline in chronic diseases such as breast cancer and a restoration of vitality and youthfulness: 1) hormones must be balanced, preferably with bio-identical versions, to the levels found in one's mid-twenties; 2) the detoxification system must be restored; and 3) the body's toxic load must be reduced.

An important component of hormonal balancing is the use of estrogen, but this would be challenged by the outcome of a random controlled trial using synthetic estrogen and progestin. The premature interruption of the Women's Health Initiative (WHI) study, due to an increased risk of breast cancer for those women using the synthetic hormone preparation Prempro, threw the world of hormonal balancing into turmoil. What some had predicted now seemed to be validated by this study — "Hormone Replacement Therapy Causes Breast Cancer." The media, which have become an important source of medical information for the public, provided their own spin to the WHI conclusions. Widespread anxiety ensued, resulting in estrogen of any type being labeled as carcinogenic to the breast. Postmenopausal women abruptly stopped taking hormones either on their own accord or under the advice of their physicians. Those just entering menopause and who suffered from hormone-related debilitating symptoms were even more confused because just like their post-menopausal counterparts, they were being told to avoid estrogen replacement without being provided any reasonable alternatives.

Since no distinction had been made between the types of hormones used in the WHI study versus the bio-identical hormones used in my program, I was forced to justify bio-identical use and safety. On countless occasions, women would proclaim at their office visit: "Taking estrogen scares me because I read that it causes breast cancer." A review of almost three thousand patients' records from my own practice revealed no association between bio-identical estrogen replacement and breast cancer. Nor was there any increase in blood clots, strokes, or heart disease.

The wellness protocols applied to these women became the basis for the FEM Centre Breast Care Pyramid. Hormonal replacement including the use of bio-identical estrogen can be accomplished while avoiding breast cancer. A careful search of the medical literature supports the contention that women who are on a properly implemented estrogen replacement program are healthier, live longer, and have less overall risk for cancer.

Each level of the Breast Care Pyramid was arrived at by formulating concepts that had sound, evidence-based medical support for hormone replacement and breast care. The concepts were then merged into the FEM Centre Wellness Program and evaluated in a population of several thousand women, the majority of whom were postmenopausal and followed on a long-term basis.

The pyramid demonstrates an order of importance assigned to each wellness concept. Clinical experience has taught us that the success of each level listed in the pyramid is built upon those below it. Even though each concept has been assigned a different location, all are essential to complete the pyramid.

The basis for the success of this program is a healthy lifestyle, which includes proper exercise, stress reduction, and good nutrition. Once this has been mastered, one must remove the toxins that have accumulated in the body. (Detoxification is easier to accomplish with a healthy lifestyle already in place.) To quickly assess your toxicity level, complete the Detoxification Questionnaire in Appendix A.

After cleansing the body's filtering system, hormones can then be balanced. These include estrogen, progesterone, testosterone, DHEA, thyroid, pregnenolone, melatonin, insulin, cortisol, and human growth hormone. Many books have been written on hormonal balancing, but very few have discussed the role of detoxification in achieving this balance. Special supplements should also be considered that control cell division and create an optimal hormonal environment for the cell.

If the Breast Care Program is properly instituted there should be little need for traditional medical intervention. We do, however, advocate breast cancer screening, which includes both periodic use of thermograms and mammograms.

You may be surprised by the inclusion of Chapter 12 in this book. Why would a gynecologist discuss male wellness in a book devoted to women's health? My interest in male hormones began one day as I was sitting in one of my exam rooms discussing with a postmenopausal woman the symptoms she had suffered from for almost a year. It dawned on me that I was having similar issues, which led me to wonder whether my hormones were also out of balance.

It makes sense that men's hormones also require attention with aging, so why not use a gender-appropriate wellness program with bio-identical hormone replacement? Remember the old saying, "What is good for the goose is good for the gander"?

Because of my symptoms and the requests by many of my patients for me to help their husbands, I began to attend courses on male menopause (also called andropause or viropause). Over a period of time I used the knowledge gained from the FEM Centre's women's program and combined it with the gender-specific information obtained at these seminars to construct a FEM Centre Male Wellness Program. Implementation of this wellness program by both myself and the male partners of many of my patients resulted in a resounding improvement of symptoms.

Over a period of time it became apparent that couples who participated together in my program had better overall compliance. After all, how could a woman sustain on a long-term basis healthy eating, stress reduction, and exercise habits when her male partner either suffered from the symptoms of aging or maintained poor health habits? From this observation came the notion of becoming partners in health, and therefore, Chapter 12.

A recent television commercial has helped illustrate an important medical point addressed in the book. The commercial began with a midlife woman recalling that her 42-year-old sister, who was very concerned about breast cancer, had started mammogram screening at the age of forty and had one every year since that time. Unfortunately, the sister died at age 47 of heart disease.

Cancer and heart disease seem to be jockeying for the honor of being the number one killer of women. Heart disease has just recently been replaced by cancer. Regardless of which is first or second, the same principles used in avoiding breast cancer also apply to other cancers and even heart disease. The origin or cause is remarkably similar among all of the chronic diseases of aging. The FEM Centre Breast Care Program could be called the FEM Centre Heart, Cancer, Brain, or Bone Program.

Every attempt has been made to create a program that is effective, reasonably easy to follow, and affordable. Even if all of the suggestions cannot be implemented, it is still worth pursuing those that can be accomplished on a long-term basis.

Some of the recommendations may not be covered by health insurers. Insurance reimbursement is generally approved only for intervention rather than prevention. This practice is not limited just to health coverage; one need look no further than the automobile insurance industry, which provides for car damage but rarely preventive maintenance.

Remember that your body, unlike the car, cannot be traded in for a new model. Priorities must be established, and what is more important than your health?

CHAPTER 1

Cancer and Breast Health

Mention breast cancer, and most women shudder at the mere sound of that two-word time bomb. Thoughts of friends, sisters, mothers, aunts, cousins — a long list of past casualties or potential victims swirls in the corners of one's mind. It elicits fears, tears, unease, panic, alarm, memories of lost loved ones or simply the anxious dread of a random act of fate in which a sudden, frightening diagnosis appears out of nowhere. No one wants to hear those words. It doesn't change the reality or the statistics.

As we age, the anxiety grows because every woman knows that as the years mount, so do her chances for breast cancer. More than 80 percent of breast cancer occurs in women over the age of 50 with the median age for breast cancer diagnosis being 64 years. The chance for breast cancer for a woman of 40 is 1 in 217. By the time she is sixty it is 1 in 24.

Add to all that the recent news concerning hormone replacement therapy (HRT). Originally intended to optimize the health of pre- and postmenopausal women, we are now told HRT can increase one's chances for strokes and breast cancer. What's a woman to do?

This predicament has been caused largely by distillation of complex medical studies into simplistic sound bites for dissemination through our mass media. Reporters and editors (many of whom have little or no medical training) are forced to reduce the often extensive protocols and findings of these studies into 30- to 45-second "medical alerts" on television, or 200-word "medical news" stories in the newspaper. Short on information but long on angst, these often distorted reports only contribute to the fear and confusion a woman faces.

I am sure you have seen or heard such "breaking news" as:

"Hormone Replacement Therapy Increases Cancer Risk!"
"Study Shows Estrogen's Role in Cancer, Stroke, Heart Disease"
"Study Recommends Women Avoid Hormone Replacement "

Thus, the contemporary woman is faced with this apparent dilemma:

1. Using HRT to help get through pre- and postmenopause all the while raising the risk of breast cancer, stroke, and heart disease, or

2. Avoiding these increased risks but suffering through hot flashes, never-ending headaches, fuzzy memory, fatigue, mood swings, and uncontrolled weight gain.

It doesn't have to be this way. With this book I hope to:

- Ease your fears.

- Help you avoid the negative effects of pre- and postmenopause while maintaining the health of your breasts.

- Optimize your overall health, especially that of your breasts, whether or not you use hormone replacement therapy.

- Minimize your risks for developing breast cancer.

These are important goals, first, because balancing your hormones and alleviating menopausal symptoms will not only improve your daily life but your long-term health as well. Second, avoiding breast cancer is preferable to treating it once it occurs.

As we all know, cancer treatment is difficult and can have many profound and damaging effects. Chemotherapy is but one obvious example of the cure being nearly as bad as the disease. There are others that are even grimmer to bear.

Most breast cancer organizations arrive too late. These associations are "support" oriented. They concentrate on helping a woman deal with breast cancer once it has occurred and focus little on significant research dedicated to prevention.

There are groups geared toward research and education relative to treatment, therapies and screening procedures, but the pharmaceutical industry is the primary controller of cancer research, either directly or through the administration of grants. The interests of pharmaceutical companies are obviously focused on treatment versus prevention because of the greater potential for a return on their corporate investments. Unfortunately, this control also stifles research on natural and botanical supplements since they are in the "public domain" and can't be patented and brought to market with high profit margins.

Through the natural chemistry and biology of the plant world, many methods and substances have developed that control cell division to prevent tumorous growths. It is my belief that we should be able to take advantage of nature's own inherent knowledge of chemical and biological processes that have evolved through trial and error over millions of years. I use many such natural, plant-based substances as key ingredients in the FEM Centre Breast Care Program.

This is not a cancer "treatment," but a preventive aid. The FEM Centre Breast Care Program is based on medical literature and clinical experience. The program integrates information from randomly controlled trials with the insight of complementary medicine and a thorough understanding of the intricacies of hormones and how they work throughout the body. The goal is to decrease your risk for breast cancer and encourage a positive, healthy lifestyle.

Obviously, there can be no guarantees when dealing with breast cancer. However, the sooner you start the FEM Centre program, the sooner your risk will begin to diminish. And the longer you stick to it, the more you will increase the health of your breasts and the overall well-being of your heart, bones, brain, and digestive system.

Breast cancer takes approximately seven to ten years to go from a cell to a level that is detectable by various screening methods. This means that by the time medical treatment intervenes, the cancer has had a decade or so to do its work.

The good news — despite what you've heard from the media — is that you *can* continue with hormone replacement therapy without jeopardizing the health of your breasts. Or you can dispense with HRT, and our program will still help your breasts by providing preventive measures to minimize your risk of breast cancer.

One thing I must emphasize: This is a long-term program and the results will be mostly unseen, although weight loss combined with an increased overall feeling of wellness are likely to be noticeable effects of the program.

CHAPTER 2

Causes of Breast Cancer

The cancer epidemic is relatively recent in origin and appears to be a unique by-product of our modern industrial age. At the beginning of the 20th century, 41,000 Americans died of cancer each year — a rate of approximately 64 per 100,000. By 1990, the death rate per 100,000 was nearly three times the 1900 figure. By the mid-1990s, 1,250,000 Americans were diagnosed with cancer and were dying at an average rate of 1,550 per day. Cancer has replaced heart disease as the number one killer of Americans under the age of eighty-five.

In the 19th century, breast cancer was a comparatively rare occurrence. According to the American Cancer Society an estimated 215,000 women in the United States will be diagnosed with breast cancer in 2005.

What changed so much in the last 100 years? Did the industrial and technological "progress" of this century play a part? What can we do to reverse the trend?

To be able to answer these questions, we need to understand the process by which cancer arises.

First, there are two phases breast cells must pass through in order to develop into a clinically detectable malignancy. These are known as *initiation* and *propagation*. Initiation is where a specific agent causes a single cell to become a cancer cell. Propagation is the promotion of excessive cell division — or the growth of a cancer tumor.

Second, there seems to be no one cause or initiator to which breast cancer can be attributed, but more likely a combination of factors push a cell into dividing uncontrollably without regard for neighboring cells.

Note: An estrogen imbalance within breast cells can act both as an initiator and a propagator. FEM Centre's Breast Care Program, which stresses prevention, minimizes the occurrence of both.

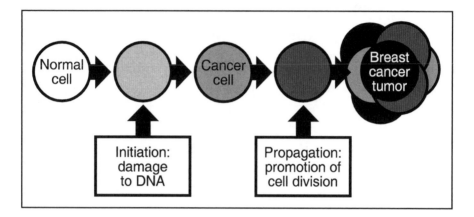

Figure 1. *The cancer-initiation-to-cancer-propagation path. Once a cell has become malignant, propagation (increased cell division) occurs.*

Researchers believe that cancer can be initiated in two ways:

1. Changing the cell's genetic blueprint, by actual damage or by random chance (mutation).
2. Damage to the supporting structure that encases the cell (known as the cell matrix).

DNA Damage

Each of your breast cells relies on DNA to provide proper and accurate instructions for its operation. DNA is a complex molecular protein in the nucleus of the cell that contains the genetic blueprint directing the cell's function. It tells the cell what duties to perform, how to perform them, and when to divide. If the blueprint becomes damaged, the breast cell can receive inaccurate operating instructions resulting in either premature cell death or cell malfunction leading to uncontrolled division.

Free radicals are electrically charged molecules that damage the DNA by disrupting its structure. A wide variety of elements including diet, a sedentary lifestyle, environmental pollution, radiation, and even hormonal imbalances can increase the concentration of free radicals in the body. Free radicals are thought to damage breast cell DNA, thus initiating the formation of cancer cells. Even more disturbing, genetic variations inherited from your parents can amplify the damage free radicals do to DNA.

Some researchers believe one reason we grow old is through the accumulation of damaged DNA. What we do know is that the amount of damaged DNA increases with age, as does the incidence of cancer.

The program described in this book will show you how to lower the risk of DNA injury, decreasing your risk of breast cancer.

Cell Matrix Damage

Traditional medicine has focused primarily on cellular function as the origin of disease. However, the neighborhood in which a breast cell resides can initiate malignant growths independent of damage to the DNA.

Research has shown that the matrix surrounding and holding the cells together may be the most important determinant of not only susceptibility to breast cancer, but overall health as well. In contrast to the rigid structure of a cell, the cell matrix is one of the most dynamic areas of the body. It consists of a collagen/glycoprotein glue that contains nerves, lymphatic channels, and small blood vessels (capillaries) that support and nourish the cells. Toxins such as heavy metals, pesticides, and free radicals accumulate in this matrix and eventually undermine its integrity. Disturbing this matrix can result in uncontrolled cell division or the initiation of cancer.

Investigational data indicate that apparently normal breast cells with intact DNA can become cancerous when transplanted into tissue whose matrix has been damaged by radiation. Much like a seed surrounded by soil, it is the condition of the matrix that helps determine whether a cancer "seed" can flourish.

In order for your breast, heart, brain, bone, and trillions of other cells that make up your body to function their best and protect against disease, the health of the cellular matrix must be addressed through *detoxification* — a cleansing and restoration of the cell matrix — detailed in Chapter 8 of this book.

Risk Factors

Diet and Pollution

Drastic changes in our diet over the last century, biologic additives introduced into our food supply, and the omnipresent pollutants in our environment all contribute to our current breast cancer epidemic.

Food is the most important and powerful medicine you can take. It is less expensive than drugs and doesn't require a prescription from your doctor. Food works with your body's natural defenses to guard against disease and aids in the body's repair during and after a disease or injury.

The right foods can make all the difference — supporting your internal systems, boosting your energy level, and extending your life span. On the other hand, the wrong foods can do just the opposite. For example, cancers and heart disease occur more frequently in countries with a high intake of saturated fat.

Even the preparation of food can be important. Foods that are blackened or charred over an open flame can create chemicals that are carcinogenic.

Beyond that, most foods in our supermarkets are polluted with man-made chemical additives, pesticides sprayed on fruits, grains and vegetables, and antibiotics used in animal stock destined for our tables. The common practice of removing essential vitamins and fiber has led to the emergence of unhealthy "processed" foods. And finally, we face introduction of genetically engineered foods, of which there is little knowledge about the long-term effects. This list comprises but a few of the many suspicious changes in what was once a stable, wholesome diet for thousands of years.

The environmental pollutants we come into contact with on a daily basis, many being inherently carcinogenic, can also have dramatic effects on the body. Many plastics used in the packaging of our foods and beverages and molded into toys for our children leach toxic substances that can't be seen, smelled, or tasted. Toxins like cadmium, mercury, lead, and arsenic pollute our air, food, and water, finding their way into our bodies and affecting our internal systems, our organs, our cells, and our DNA.

Radiation exposure also seems to increase the likelihood of developing breast cancer in the long term. For example, a study shows that women who received radiation therapy for treatment of Hodgkin's disease before age 15 have a significantly higher rate of breast cancer than the general population.

There is not enough data to precisely identify the many complex relationships between diet, environmental toxins, and breast cancer, but there is enough scientific evidence to conclude that such relationships exist, and that making a few important alterations to your diet and lifestyle can profoundly reduce your risk for breast cancer. In short, putting *good* food into the body and reducing toxins via detoxification can be a positive, proactive method of improving your health and extending your life.

Genetics

Genetics is another important element in determining breast cancer risk. A family history of breast cancer is a well-documented risk factor, and the risk is highest if the affected relative developed breast cancer at a young age or if she is a close relative such as a mother, sister, daughter, or aunt.

There is a great deal of research on genes linked to breast cancer, and recent findings have helped isolate a few important genetic suspects. BRCA1 is a gene that controls the rate of breast cell division. A mutated BRCA1 gene markedly increases the threat of breast cancer to a lifetime risk of almost 85 percent, plus, women who have this mutated BRCA1 gene tend to develop breast cancer at an early age. Women with this genetic abnormality also have an increased likelihood of developing ovarian cancer. BRCA2 is a second gene that if mutated can increase the risk of developing breast cancer but not necessarily ovarian cancer.

Only those women who have a strong family history of breast cancer are counseled to be tested for these genes. The issues surrounding genetic testing are complicated, and women who are interested should discuss this with their health care providers.

Having said this, it is also important to say — breast cancer doesn't discriminate! Between 80 and 85 percent of all breast cancers occur in women who have no family history of the disease, while other women tend to underestimate their risk because it hasn't appeared in their family in a generation or two. This is a mistake!

Other genes are also important in the prevention of breast cancer. These genes assist in detoxification; formation and inactivation of estrogen metabolites; and providing receptors for vitamin D — just to name a few of their functions. With the mapping of the human genome, specialty labs can now offer blood tests that can identify those women who have miscoded genes. These damaged genes inhibit normal chemical reactions, increasing the initiation and propagation steps in the development of breast cancer. By uncovering these problems in advance, one can maximize the advantages of our breast care program.

Hormonal History

Your hormonal history can play an important role in the development of breast cancer. Women who start menstruating at an early age or experience a late menopause have a higher risk of breast cancer. Conversely, beginning menstrual periods at an older age and experiencing early menopause tend to offer protection from breast cancer. Having a child before age 30 may provide some protection as well, while having no children may increase risk for developing breast cancer.

Oral Contraceptives

The association between breast cancer and oral contraceptives is controversial. While studies have shown that long-term use of oral contraceptives produces no significant increased risk for breast cancer, there seems to be a small group of younger women whose use for more than four years results in a higher risk for breast cancer before age 45. With relatively inconclusive data on this subject, the importance of pregnancy prevention versus the long-term health of the breasts must be carefully considered. Should one decide to use the birth control pill, I suggest routine breast thermograms (see Chapter 11). It is also important to point out that since the final maturation of the breasts occurs in pregnancy, a full-term gestation and subsequent breast-feeding contribute to a lower risk of breast cancer.

CHAPTER 3

Estrogen Explained

Estrogen has a major impact on some three hundred of your tissue systems helping you to stay young, energetic, and healthy. One of its main functions is to stimulate sensitive cells (uterus and breast) to undergo mitosis or cell division. A proper balance of estrogen enhances sensuality, brings a glow to the skin, moisturizes the eyes, lubricates the vagina, gives fullness to the breasts, preserves clarity of thought, and protects the bones and cardiovascular system. This miraculous product of nature shapes mind, body, and emotions. It wields great power over every aspect of mental and physical health, so it is important to keep it in a perfect, natural balance.

Before adolescence, male and female breasts are alike. But once females near puberty — before menstruation begins — estrogen triggers their transition from child to adult. It is literally what makes you a woman. (In addition, progesterone, insulin, thyroid hormone, prolactin, and human growth hormone are required for maturation of the breasts.)

The breast has been described as resembling a thick forest. The interwoven limbs and vines of that forest are a complex web of connective tissue, nerves, blood vessels, and lymph nodes. Using this analogy, an individual "tree" is the main milk duct, with branches being smaller milk ducts, and finally, the "leaves" representing the clusters of milk-producing glands called alveoli, which make up the mammary lobe. Each alveolus is lined by a single layer of cells which, when stimulated by hormones, secrete milk. After entering the alveolus, the milk is propelled through the ductal system (lactiferous duct) and finally is expressed at the opening of the nipple.

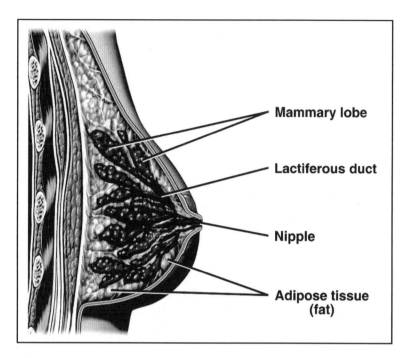

Figure 2. Anatomy of the breast.

The alveoli, contained in the mammary lobes, and the lactiferous ducts are the hormone-sensitive regions of the breast. Ducts seem to require only estrogen to grow, while alveoli need both estrogen and progesterone to mature. (It is abnormal cell division in either of these two breast structures — intraductal in the ducts, or lobular in the alveoli — that results in breast cancer.)

During the teenage years, the breasts are very dense and predominately glandular. As one ages, this glandular tissue is replaced by fat. After menopause, this process accelerates so that by the time one reaches their sixties, most of the glandular tissue has been replaced by fat.

In premenopause, an estrogen imbalance such as excess estrogen (estrogen dominance) can occur. The breast is subjected to higher levels of estrogen. This intense exposure can cause excessive cell division leading to fibrocystic breast disease. Almost 80 percent of women at some point in their lives eventually experience at least microscopic fibrocystic changes. These changes are painful and worrisome and have been shown to increase the relative risk of subsequent breast cancer twofold. Estrogen dominance can also result in irritable moods, swelling, bloating, breast tenderness, heavy menstrual flows, uterine fibroids, and endometriosis.

Conversely, estrogen deficiency (generally referred to as menopause) gives rise to hot flashes, night sweats, fatigue, fuzzy memory, insomnia, depression, osteoporosis, bladder urgency, and an increase in susceptibility to the chronic diseases of aging such as heart disease.

Note: Since it acts to nourish nerve cells while increasing levels of the mood elevating neurotransmitter serotonin, estrogen is also a hormone of the brain. With the startling increase in Alzheimer's disease coupled with the increase in female life expectancy, a healthy brain is of utmost importance to a successful anti-aging program. One in four women will contract Alzheimer's by age eighty. The average age of onset is almost ten years earlier than in men, and an additional three years earlier if a woman's ovaries have been surgically removed. For those who take estrogen for at least six months, some studies show, the risk diminishes by 60 percent.

The Three Types of Internally Produced Estrogens

Estrogen is a generic term generally applied to the three natural, internally produced molecules: estrone (E1), estradiol (E2), and estriol (E3).

Estrone is the predominate estrogen found in postmenopause, and is thought by some to contribute to an increased risk of breast cancer in postmenopausal women (although I believe this to be erroneous). When estrone is in its most common form, estrone sulfate, it cannot enter the breast cell. This prevents the overstimulation of the cell, minimizing the possible formation of cancer.

Estradiol (the most powerful of the three natural estrogens) is made mainly by the ovaries prior to menopause. The majority of postmenopausal production of estradiol occurs in individual cells throughout the body, especially fat cells and stromal cells in the breast. When a doctor tries to measure postmenopausal estradiol, the ratio of estradiol in the breast cell to that in the blood can vary by huge amounts (up to 20 times), which is meant only to illustrate that measuring hormonal levels using blood or saliva does not accurately reflect what is present inside the cells.

Estriol (the weakest of the natural estrogens) in its active form is found in significant quantities in the blood only during pregnancy, when it is made by the placenta. In the non-pregnant woman it is primarily found as biologically inactive estriol, which is derived from the breakdown of estradiol and estrone in the liver.

If administered in large enough quantities, the active form of estriol can stimulate the uterine lining to grow and breast cells to divide. Estriol also has been shown to have a protective effect against breast cancer and is frequently used in breast cancer survivors who desire estrogen replacement therapy.

The amount of estrogen in the postmenopausal breast can be accounted for primarily by the amount 1) recycled from the intestines, and 2) manufactured by both fat and breast cells.

Recycled estrogen is estrogen that is meant to be excreted from the body by the intestines but is instead reabsorbed into the bloodstream. The decreased function of this finely tuned disposal mechanism results from poor bowel function, excess activity of the enzyme beta-glucuronidase, and inadequate detoxification by the liver.

In postmenopausal women, adrenal hormones like DHEA are the main building blocks required by breast and fat cells to manufacture estrone and estradiol. This process does not depend upon the estrogen that you receive from bio-identical replacement therapy; instead it is controlled by the activity of certain enzymes (such as aromatase and 17β-hydroxysteroid dehydrogenase). Your genetic makeup and diet determine how efficiently these enzymes work.

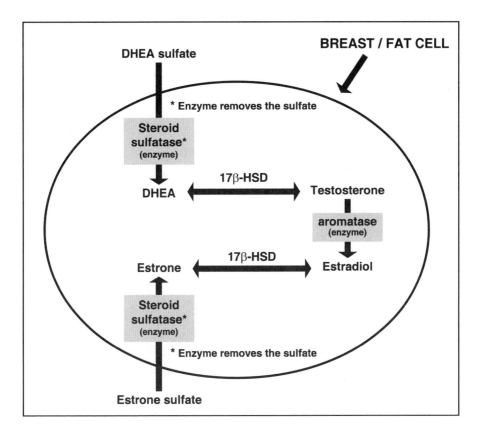

Figure 3. *The effects of 17β-HSD and aromatase on the production of estradiol in the breast and fat cell.*

Figure 3 illustrates the three enzymatic stages involved in the formation of estradiol inside fat and breast cells. Nutritional substances are capable of controlling these stages, thus preventing the overproduction of estradiol. Excessive activity of steroid sulfatase, 17β-hydroxysteroid dehydrogenase (17β-HSD), and aromatase has been shown to be a risk factor for breast cancer. This pathway is also thought to be important in the etiology of prostate cancer.

Stage One

Stage One begins with the attachment of a sulfate molecule to either estrogen or DHEA (sulfation). This chemical process allows molecules to become water-soluble and then be transported throughout the body. Sulfation also biologically inactivates hormones so that they cannot enter the cell or attach to its receptors. Once the sulfated hormone (DHEAS or estrone sulfate) has been delivered to the cell, a sulfatase enzyme (whose action is the opposite of sulfation) is required to remove the sulfate molecule activating the hormone and allowing it to enter into the pathway described in Figure 3. Research has shown that the pathway leading to the removal of the sulfate molecule is one hundred to five hundred times more active than the Stage 3 or aromatase pathway. Should the sulfatase enzyme become overactive, it would flood the cell with too much bioactive DHEA or estrone and lead to excessive production of estradiol. Testosterone, progesterone, and 2-methoxyestrogen (the methylated form of the 2-hydroxyestrogen) protect the breast cell by slowing the steroid sulfatase process.

Estradiol, at levels much higher than normally found in the body, can inhibit the breast cell from dividing. High-dose estrogen therapy is even used to treat advanced cases of breast cancer. This apparent paradox is known as the "Janus effect." According to roman mythology, Janus was the god of doorways and gates who was depicted as having two faces pointed in opposite directions. One face of estrogen, especially at those low to moderate levels found in a woman's hormonal transitions, is to promote cell division while the other face of estrogen is to inhibit division at much higher levels. A mechanism that could possibly explain this inhibition of cell division is the surprising ability of estradiol to block the sulfatase reaction.

The Janus effect may also account for the decrease in breast cancer rates among those women who used only Premarin in the Women's Health Initiative study and the lack of increased recurrence in breast cancer survivors on estrogen replacement. In the *Journal of the National Cancer Institute*, Dr. Song has reported that when hormone-dependent breast cancer cells have been deprived of estradiol for an extended period of time (such as that seen in a postmenopausal woman), reintroduction of estradiol not only stops these cells from dividing but can induce programmed cell death, or apoptosis.

Stage Two

17β-HSD mediates the conversion of DHEA to testosterone and estrone to estradiol. This enzyme has been called the intracellular switch, which controls the hormonal environment of the breast cell. Progesterone and vitamin D prevent its overreactivity.

Stage Three

Stage three involves the conversion of testosterone into estradiol by the enzymatic reaction of aromatase. Red wine extract, 2-methoxyestrogen, and specific drugs (Femara, Aromasin, Arimidex) used in treating breast cancer act to inhibit aromatase.

It is easy to see from Figure 3 how excessive amounts of fat can contribute to hormonal imbalance and overstimulation of the breast cells through the release of 17β-HSD-derived estrogens into the bloodstream.

Note: The FEM Centre Breast Care Program provides for the regulation of these enzymes in order to create a suitable hormonal environment for the postmenopausal breast cell. It follows the Breast Care Pyramid detailed in Chapter 6.

The Externally Produced Estrogens

In addition to the internally produced estrogens, four different types of externally produced estrogens can affect your health:

- Bio-identical (or native) estrogens

- Synthetic estrogens

- Xenoestrogens

- Phytoestrogens

Bio-identical (native) estrogens are considered to be natural hormones. Bio-identical estrogens are generally derived from plants and have the exact same structure as the hormones made by the human body. Yes, they are identical. They are ideal for use in hormone replacement therapy and — because they are natural — are recommended by the FEM Centre Breast Care Program.

Synthetic estrogens, in particular those that are chemically manipulated, are known as *non-identical* hormones. The molecular structure of synthetics is very different from human/bio-identical estrogens.

In the synthetic category are widely used products that can have negative effects on your health. Premarin and Prempro are popular compounds containing synthetic estrogen manufactured from the urine of pregnant horses. Needless to say, a woman's metabolism differs significantly from that of the average mare!

These non-identical hormones, scientists have found, bind to cell receptors differently than natural hormones and tended to accumulate in the body. Consequently, breast cell metabolism is inappropriately stimulated, and the cell's genetic material is damaged, potentially leaving a woman using the hormones at a higher risk of breast cancer, blood clots, heart disease, and other illnesses.

Xenoestrogens are the third category of externally produced hormones. They are perhaps the most hazardous of all. Xenoestrogens (literally, "foreign" estrogens) are produced as by-products of our overpolluted world. They are in our food, air, and water. They can be absorbed through your skin, inhaled by the lungs, and ingested when you eat.

Examples include dioxins and other organochlorine elements with long names such as: dichlorodiphenyl-trichloroethane (DDT), polychlorinated biphenyls (PCB), and 2,3,7,8,tetrachlorodibenzo-p-dioxin (TCDD). Xenoestrogens can be stored in fat cells and can remain there for long periods of time. Although relatively weak (1/5,000th to 1/1,000,000th the strength of estradiol), they can act in combination to have a cancer-causing effect on the breast by: 1) increasing the enzyme that favors the formation of 4-hydroxyestrogen (see Chapter 4) and 2) providing low-grade estrogen stimulation to the breast cell.

Synthetic estrogens in the presence of xenoestrogens are especially dangerous. This toxic soup can result in hormonal overstimulation of the breast cell, leading to genetic damage and eventually to cancer.

Phytoestrogens are labeled according to chemical structure: lignans, isoflavones, and coumestans. Lignans are found in cereals, vegetables, legumes, green tea, and fruit, with the highest concentrations being found in oilseed such as flax. Isoflavones occur in soy products, beer, legumes, chickpeas, beans, and lentils. Coumestrol is present in grapes (resveratrol), alfalfa, clover, and mungbeans.

Their effect on the breast has generated a great deal of attention while leading to misconceptions. They are not really hormones and do not closely resemble estrogen structures, yet these plant-derived compounds, abundant in nature, can weakly interact with an estrogen receptor. While the weakest of the natural estrogens, estriol, has about 1/80th the binding capacity of estradiol, phytoestrogens have approximately 1/500th to 1/10,000th the binding capacity, and have been shown in some studies to stimulate the growth of breast cancer cells.

Does this mean that foods such as soy and flax lead to breast cancer? Upon examining women in Asia and Japan who eat soy on a daily basis, we find that phytoestrogens (usually 25 to 45 milligrams of isoflavones daily) have a protective effect.

This contradiction between experiments and observation is explained by the fact that phytoestrogens, in addition to weakly binding with the estrogen receptors, also inhibit the production of estrogen. Eating a diet rich in phytoestrogens has been shown to lower estrogen levels in women. The resulting lowered levels *protect* against breast cancer.

The biologically active forms of certain phytoestrogens are formed during the digestion process. After you consume a phytoestrogen, such as soy, the good bacteria in your colon convert it into its bioactive form, which is absorbed by the intestine and later eliminated from the body either in the urine or by the intestines. Soy is metabolized into daidzein and genistein. In some women, daidzein can be further converted to equol, which has been shown to be protective against breast disease.

Note: If you take antibiotics, the good bacteria in the intestines are destroyed, preventing the conversion of phytoestrogens to their protective metabolites.

Phytoestrogens such as soy isoflavones can be considered as *adaptogenic*. When estrogen levels are elevated, soy seems to compete with the stronger estrogen for receptor sites, lowering the total estrogen effect. Conversely, if estrogen levels are low, such as in postmenopause, soy isoflavones help fill the empty receptor sites, raising the estrogen effect.

Soy is a common, multipurpose food source that contains phytoestrogens along with fiber, protein, and plant sterols. Several studies have shown the protective effects of soy on the breast. Premenopausal women and those who metabolize soy into equol seemed to be afforded the greatest protection (but only 30 percent of women have the necessary enzyme in the colon to synthesize equol from soy). Other studies have demonstrated that moderate soy consumption in breast cancer survivors is safe. There have also been reports linking excessive ingestion of soy with thyroid abnormalities (usually at doses greater than 120 mg of isoflavones daily).

I suggest moderate consumption of soy (if possible, in a fermented form) on a rotational basis. The amount of soy that should be consumed is determined by the total daily dose of isoflavones — 30 to 70 milligrams per day. To avoid the development of sensitivities or allergies, never use soy as the sole protein source, but always rotate it with other food sources.

In addition, flaxseed is a lignan-phytoestrogen that we highly recommend because of its breast-protective effects. Flaxseed contains the omega-3 fatty acid — alpha linolenic acid. However, this particular form of omega-3 is not readily converted by your body into the more powerful EPA (eicosapentaenoic acid) and DHA (docosahexaenoic acid). While there is some evidence that alpha linolenic acid lowers the risk of breast cancer, I believe that it is the lignans contained in the flaxseed itself that provides the protection. These lignans increase the production of the beneficial 2-hydroxyestrogens.

Studies have shown that daily intake of 5 to 10 grams of freshly ground flaxseed optimizes estrogen metabolites while regulating bowel function.

Resveratrol, a form of coumestrol-phytoestrogen, is found in red grape skins. It is an essential part of the FEM Center Breast Care Program and explained in Chapter 10 — Breast Care Nutrients.

The hormonal environment of the postmenopausal breast cell is influenced by the amount of estrogen derived from both internal and external sources. Your externally produced estrogen load is controlled by the degree of exposure to phytoestrogens in your diet, xenoestrogens that pollute your environment, and the amount and type of estrogen replacement you use.

However, because your breasts manufacture estrogen, the amount of bio-identical estrogen you receive in hormone therapy is not necessarily as important as how your body converts and utilizes it. In other words, "It's not what you take, it's what you make."

Still, women can favorably influence internal and external estrogen exposure, minimizing possible damage to your breast cells. With its emphasis on stress reduction, good dietary choices, detoxification, and hormonal balancing, the FEM Centre Breast Care Pyramid can show you how.

CHAPTER 4

Estrogen and the WHI Study

Scientific studies on the effects of hormone replacement therapy (HRT) after menopause have had conflicting results and conclusions. The most prominent, publicized, and confusing study for consumers was the recent one by the Women's Health Initiative (WHI). Many physicians use the WHI study as a guide in determining the role of estrogen replacement in their patients. In most cases this translates to: *avoid* hormone replacement therapy. However, I believe the study is more of a guide on "what not to do" than a denunciation of HRT.

Findings from this research, along with a handful of other contemporary studies, are not well understood by the average person (and many physicians), therefore, it is time to examine the facts surrounding this controversial study.

The Women's Health Initiative study was a randomized, controlled study using orally administered synthetic hormones. Prempro was used if the woman had a uterus and Premarin was used for those who had undergone a hysterectomy.

Prempro is a combination of two synthetic hormones, Provera (a synthetic progestin) and Premarin (a horse-derived estrogen), and was chosen because it is the one most commonly prescribed for women receiving hormone replacement therapy. It is important to state that this study *did not* use bio-identical estrogens or progesterone, which are the ideal types of hormones and the ones we recommend. In addition, no consideration was given to lifestyle (smoking vs. non-smoking), diet, exercise, hormonal balance, and detoxification, all critical components of a healthy and effective breast care program.

Note: It has been said that before age 40, our body takes care of itself; after 40, we must take care of our bodies. I believe this to be true, and a good example is a recent estimate that after age 40, we're able to influence 75 percent of our genetic tendencies merely by making proper lifestyle decisions (such as quitting smoking, getting more exercise, and choosing a healthy diet).

The most widely publicized finding from the WHI study said that estrogen hormone treatment increases the chances of heart disease, stroke, and breast cancer. In fact, the Prempro portion of the study was abruptly canceled due to these increased risks. Remember, this part of the study used synthetic progestin (Provera) combined with synthetic estrogen (Premarin).

The Premarin leg of the study showed that women had less breast cancer on Premarin than if they were on no hormones at all (the Janus effect)! There was still an increased risk of blood clots and strokes, however. This indicates that the combination of synthetic hormones (Provera and Premarin) may pose a greater risk for breast cancer than just the synthetic estrogen alone, although as emphasized earlier, all synthetic hormones are to be avoided in favor of bio-identical versions.

To properly understand the results of the WHI and various other recent studies, it's important to make some distinctions about estrogen, which also requires a bit of background information about the way estrogen works. First we will look at how estrogen and the products of its metabolism (metabolites) affect cells, sometimes by latching onto "receptors" much the way a lock fits a key.

How Does Estrogen Interact with the Breast Cell?

The biologic effects of estrogen on the breast cell include:

- The binding of estrogen and its metabolites with the estrogen receptor that resides either in the cell wall or more commonly on the membrane of the nucleus;

- The later action of subsequent metabolites of estrogen, namely 2-hydroxy, 4-hydroxy, and 16alpha-hydroxy-estrogen, which can act on the cell independently of receptors.

Hormones such as estrogen relay their messages by binding to specific breast cell receptors. After estrogen binds to a receptor on the nuclear membrane, the breast cell is stimulated to divide. As the breast cell divides, its genetic code, or DNA, is duplicated in order to form two cells that are genetically identical (mitosis). Because of the complexity of DNA, continued rapid cell division increases the chance for the DNA to be incorrectly copied, leading to a cancerous cell.

To make sure cells do not divide unchecked, normal cells, both ductal and alveolar, must self-terminate. Obviously breast health is most favorably achieved by ensuring that cells self-terminate in a timely manner and avoid being in a state of uncontrolled division (cancer).

The role of estrogen, especially synthetic versions, in the propagation of breast cancer is linked to unnecessary breast cell division. Interestingly, only about 17 percent of breast cells have an estrogen receptor. These cells are known as ER+ cells. (Those without receptors are ER– cells.) This means that a majority of breast cells do not respond to estrogen stimulation. However, if a breast cell does have estrogen receptors and has already turned malignant, estrogen can cause this cancer cell to divide even faster than those without the receptors. In fact, almost two-thirds of all breast cancers are ER+ and only one-third are ER–.

Traditional medicine has focused almost solely on the hormone-receptor binding while ignoring the non-receptor effects of the hormonal metabolites of estrogen. Our program takes both of these into account so that breast health can be achieved while using bio-identical hormone replacement therapy.

Each of the body's three estrogens — estrone, estradiol, and estriol — interacts differently with estrogen receptors. The stronger a particular estrogen binds with the receptor (the better the key fits the lock) the more the cell will be stimulated.

In the case of the breast cell, the stronger the binding of hormone to receptor, the more times the cell divides. Estradiol binds the strongest. By comparison, estrone's binding strength is only one-twelfth of that, and estriol is just one-eightieth. If there is an excessive amount of estradiol, the breast cells will continue to divide and not get a chance to rest. We describe this as *overstimulation* — a common occurrence during a woman's hormonal transitions. Symptoms of overstimulation can lead to fibrocystic changes that manifest as breast tenderness and enlargement. Other gynecologic conditions that result from overstimulation include endometriosis and fibroids.

Certain metabolites of estrogen, particularly 16alpha-hydroxy, also display a strong attraction to estrogen receptor sites. Elevations of this hormone have been found to be a breast cancer risk factor in women, especially those in perimenopause.

Popularly prescribed synthetic estrogens such as Premarin and its metabolites, equilin and dihydroequilin, attach to the estrogen receptor more firmly than estradiol. Excessive stimulation also occurs because the synthetic estrogen stays in the body longer since it lacks the enzymes necessary for timely inactivation and subsequent removal of these estrogens.

The Three Kinds of Estrogen Metabolites

As noted earlier, one of the main oversights of traditional medicine that led to the outcomes in the WHI study is the misconception that all estrogens, whether bio-identical or synthetic, have the same effect on the breast. The effects of estrogen's metabolites on breast cells are also overlooked.

As shown in Figure 4 on page 31, estrogen either enters or is produced inside the breast cell, it is eventually broken down into metabolites which themselves must eventually be removed from the body either by the kidneys or the intestine. These metabolites are:

- **2-hydroxyestrogen (2OH)** — in its methylated form (2-methoxyestrogen), kills breast cancer cells

- **4-hydroxyestrogen (4OH)** — an initiator of breast cancer; not dependent upon estrogen-receptor interaction

- **16alpha-hydroxyestrogen (16OH)** — promotes or increases breast cancer cell division; dependent mainly on estrogen-receptor interaction

The **2-hydroxyestrogen** metabolite is formed in cells such as breast and liver and has proven anti-cancer qualities. After undergoing the chemical reaction known as methylation, this metabolite inhibits rapid and abnormal cell division. It also decreases the activity of major estrogen receptors and inhibits the enzyme aromatase, limiting the amount of estradiol in the breast cell. 2-hydroxy reaches very high levels during pregnancy, which suggests it serves in a protective role against extreme hormonal elevations. Researchers have also shown that 2-hydroxy may help protect the heart, since it prevents the overgrowth of cells that line the blood vessels.

There are early indications in some studies that 2-hydroxy might be as effective as some chemotherapy medications against both ER+ and ER– breast cancers. Laboratory animals with breast tumors were given 2-hydroxy, and in many cases, the tumors shrank.

Yes, strangely enough, the breast is able to make an estrogen that actually kills breast cancer cells. This cancer-killing ability provides another reason *not* to use synthetic progestins, because they can reduce the formation of 2-hydroxyestrogens.

Levels of 2-hydroxyestrogen can be assessed by blood and urine tests. At the FEM Centre we have been able to show dramatic improvement in these levels by incorporating our recommended nutritional supplements (see Chapter 10).

4-hydroxyestrogen is also made in the breast cell. This form of estrogen metabolite has a negative tendency — it can be turned into a *mutagen*, something that tends to damage DNA. Damaged DNA can lead to mutations in the cell, causing abnormal cell division and possibly cancer.

Studies have shown that breast cancer cells have a higher level of 4-hydroxy (almost four times) when compared with 2-hydroxy. It is not possible to measure blood or urine levels of 4-hydroxyestrogen accurately because once formed, it almost instantaneously reacts with and damages the cell DNA.

Synthetic estrogens are also metabolized into 4-hydroxy products. Premarin is converted into 4-hydroxyequilenin, which is almost thirty times more toxic (or mutagenic) than those products derived from the body's own 4-hydroxyestrogens. Certainly this is a compelling reason to avoid synthetic estrogens, and a point that should have been considered in the WHI study.

The role of 4-hydroxyestrogens may not be limited just to breast cancer, but also may be found in gynecologic problems such as uterine fibroids. Fibroids are the most common tumors that occur in women and are thought to result in almost 200,000 hysterectomies in the United States yearly. Elevated levels of 4-hydroxyestrogen are found in fibroid tissue compared with normal uterine tissue. The rate of 4-hydroxyestrogen formation is almost eightfold higher in fibroid tissue than that of 2-hydroxy.

16alpha-hydroxyestrogen is made mainly in the liver. From there it enters the bloodstream and it finally comes into contact with the breast cell. Estriol, which is the weakest of the three estrogens, is derived mainly from 16alpha-hydroxyestrone. 16alpha-hydroxyestrogen acts much differently than its 4-hydroxy counterpart in that it firmly attaches to the estrogen receptor much like estradiol and causes the breast cell to rapidly divide. Again, a non-cancerous, rapidly dividing breast cell is dangerous, especially if it is subsequently injured by 4-hydroxyestrogen. In this case, it has a higher probability of becoming cancerous. Like 4-hydroxy, 16alpha-hydroxy also may have a role in DNA injury. And 16alpha-hydroxy is detected in one-third of breast tumors.

Studies have shown that 16alpha-hydroxyestrogen is important for preservation of bone tissue. That is why our breast care program uses blood testing to help ensure an optimal 2-hydroxy:16alpha-hydroxy ratio and not completely eradicate 16alpha-hydroxy.

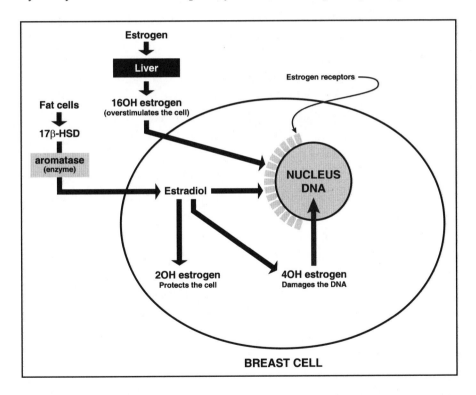

Figure 4. The different effects that 2-hydroxyestrogen, 4-hydroxyestrogen, and 16alpha-hydroxyestrogen metabolites have on the breast cell.

The WHI study did not take into account these various downstream products of estrogen, whereas the FEM Centre Breast Care Program not only takes them into account, it encourages the production of 2-hydroxy while discouraging excessive amounts of 4-hydroxy and 16alpha-hydroxy.

Hormonal Therapy "Window of Opportunity"

Another important area ignored by these studies is what I call the hormonal therapy *window of opportunity*. When a woman reaches menopause or post-menopause, there is a five- to ten-year period when the body experiences chronic inflammation. Estrogen tends to quell this inflammatory process.

As a powerful biologic fire extinguisher, estrogen can: 1) block the formation of chronic inflammatory mediators such as nuclear factor-κB (NF-κB), interleukin-6 (IL-6), tumor necrosis factor alpha (TNF-α), and prostaglandin E2 (PE2), which play important roles in the promotion of cancer, heart disease, arthritis, bone loss, and dementia; 2) promote the synthesis of endothelial nitrous oxide, which relaxes blood vessels and normalizes the blood pressure; and 3) increase a cell's sensitivity to insulin. It would take at least five to six pharmaceutical drugs to generate these beneficial effects, but, as we have seen in the past, especially with the dangers surrounding drugs such as Vioxx, synthetics rarely match those substances nature has perfected over millions of years.

If a woman enters postmenopause and does not begin any estrogen therapy within this window of opportunity (generally within the first five to ten years of postmenopause), it is difficult to begin estrogen therapy and see any prevention of chronic disease.

The average age of the women in the WHI study was sixty-three, and previous hormone therapy status was not considered among these participants. In other words, at age sixty-three, it is too late to begin estrogen therapy and expect to reverse the ravages of chronic disease, and as some studies show, the therapy could even be dangerous.

Summary: Estrogen and the WHI Study

The results of the WHI study demonstrated *what not to do* in terms of hormone balancing. In fact, this study validates our breast care program. The WHI study used single standard doses of orally administered synthetic hormones (Prempro, Premarin) instead of bio-identical versions, and showed that Prempro increased the risk of breast cancer along with increasing the risk of blood clots, strokes, and heart disease.

- The WHI study used orally administered *synthetic* hormones instead of the bio-identical versions, and showed that a combination of synthetic hormones can have dangerous side effects.

- The WHI study didn't take into account lifestyle, exercise, hormonal balance, or detoxification.

- The WHI study didn't take into account the importance of the various estrogen metabolites such as 2-hydroxy, 4-hydroxy, and 16alpha-hydroxy.

- The WHI study didn't take into account the *window of opportunity* for hormone replacement therapy and tested women who were beyond the important years for instigating hormone therapy. If a woman begins hormonal balancing early-on, from just before to shortly after menopause, she is much less likely to suffer the negative effects indicated in this study, and much more likely to see positive effects, from reducing the risk of heart disease to the prevention or reduction of the many symptoms that accompany hormonal changes.

- Most importantly, when concluded, the Premarin-only leg of the WHI revealed that women who took Premarin had a lower breast cancer rate than those who took no hormones at all (but still had an increased risk of blood clots and strokes).

CHAPTER 5

A Woman's Hormonal Transitions

The Reproductive Compartments

Endocrinologists have divided the reproductive system into compartments in order to understand how they function. Using knowledge of functional integrative medicine, I have modified these four compartmental divisions to help explain the changes the female body undergoes as hormones vary with age:

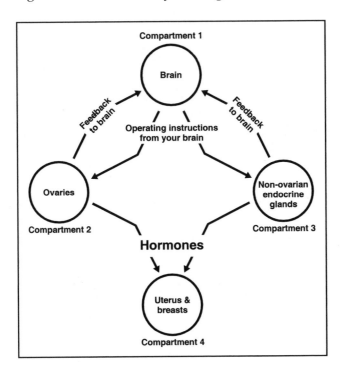

Figure 5. A woman's reproductive compartments.

1. **Brain** (composed of the higher cognitive centers, the hypothalamic areas, and the pituitary gland) — Hormonal feedback from compartments 2 and 3 help the brain determine the correct operating instructions that need to be sent out. For instance, as the ovaries begin to fail, the amount of estrogen production will decline. The brain senses this decline and releases more Follicular Stimulating Hormone level (FSH) to stimulate the ovary to increase production. Referring to Figure 7, we often find that the FSH is: 1) 10 IU/L or less but may extend into the lower teens during the reproductive and estrogen dominant transitions; 2) exceeds 10 IU/L and may climb into the upper thirties during the perimenopause; and 3) is 40 IU/L or above in menopause and postmenopause.

2. **Ovaries** — The ovaries have two important functions: ovulation (egg release by the ovary), and the production of the sex hormones estradiol, progesterone, and testosterone.

3. **Non-ovarian endocrine glands** (such as the thyroid and adrenals) — These glands are responsible for the production of hormones including DHEA, cortisol, triiodothyronine (T3) and thyroxine (T4).

4. **Uterus/Breasts** — This compartment includes the organs that are sensitive to hormones such as estrogen and play an essential role in the reproductive phase. Both the uterus and the breasts depend upon estrogen for growth and maintenance. Hormonal imbalances can have profound effects on each of these organs that may result in benign or malignant conditions. Examples include benign tumors of the uterus known as fibroids or increased intensity and frequency of menstrual flow. The breasts are subject to benign conditions such as fibrocystic changes and breast pain. Cancer can arise in the uterus or breast as a result of hormonal imbalances.

The symptoms arising from the hormonal transitions that occur with aging will be experienced differently by every woman. Some will suffer devastation, while others will breeze through without apparent problems. Understanding the dynamics and physiology that are involved in these transitions, and being properly prepared, will help you negotiate the changes discussed in this chapter.

Your future breast health begins while you are in your mother's womb and thereafter is uniquely influenced by each hormonal transition. There is no need to suffer the symptoms discussed in this chapter because of the fear that the treatment will increase your risk of breast cancer. Our program allows you to correct those imbalances that are unique to each hormonal transition while dramatically lowering the risk of breast cancer.

The goal is to extend not only life span but also health span. Even though the FEM Centre Breast Care Pyramid (see Chapter 6) should be followed throughout life, as one enters the premenopausal and postmenopausal transitions, its implementation becomes imperative in order to not only prevent breast cancer and be disease-free but to be strong, vigorous, happy, creative, and spiritually satisfied.

In order to demonstrate the complexity of your body and the evolving conditions of your hormonal status, it helps to understand the chronological history of the female physiology: adolescence, pregnancy, premenopause, menopause and the postmenopause — these are natural phases of the body as it ages. From a medical viewpoint, these changes affect each woman uniquely — the major differences being the influence of time, nature, and one's own genetics. Understanding the role that hormonal transitions play in your breast health shapes the FEM Centre Breast Care Program.

Before Birth

The first environmental exposures occur in the fetus, which is like a sponge in the mother. A fetus absorbs xenoestrogens (industrial pollutants) and heavy metals (mercury, lead, and cadmium).

Prior to pregnancy, a mother's lifestyle and nutrition set the stage for how her baby will do later in life.

Prior to pregnancy, a woman contributes to the future health of a fetus by eating the proper foods and avoiding toxins. It is important that she increase consumption of both *omega-3 fatty acids as found in fish oil*, and *folic acid* — two vital nutrients — while reducing stress and avoiding smoking and alcohol altogether.

Ancient Genes in a New World

In the early 1970s anthropologists studied tribes located in remote areas of Africa whose existence and lifestyle can be traced back to the Stone Age. The genes in your body today were really designed for the diet and lifestyle of these Stone Age tribal women.

These studies provided us with insights into the typical female hormonal transitions experienced by our early ancestors. In their hunter-gatherer environment, their diet consisted of roots, berries, and lean wild game. Due to the isolation of these tribes, they were free of our modern-day stressors and pollutants. Some of the enlightening findings of these studies included:

- Female tribal members on average first experienced menarche at 15.5 years of age. Ovulation usually began several years later, resulting in first pregnancies occurring by the late teens to early twenties.
- Frequent breast-feeding — 20 times daily — was not uncommon. The infant would sleep with the mother and suckle as needed throughout the night. Since soft foods were not readily available, breast feedings sometimes had to continue until the child was three to five years old.
- Prehistoric women had very few menstrual periods as a result of prolonged breast-feeding of the young combined with lean body mass. Their lack of excess body mass resulted from a hunter-gather diet. For a total of almost 15 years during their reproductive phase they experienced no menstrual flows. Contrast this to a modern woman, who may experience more than 200 menstrual flows in a lifetime.

There is evidence that exposure to certain toxic agents *in utero* can lead to degenerative diseases such as cancer many years later.

Mercury is an example of a very toxic agent that pregnant women can encounter without ever realizing it. Certain species of fish contain dangerous levels of mercury, but there are other places one can encounter mercury, like the dentist's office.

Mercury is a common component of dental fillings, and mercury from a mother's fillings can be partially absorbed into the bloodstream and cross the placenta, exposing the fetus to this hazardous contaminant. Mercury acts to poison the body's enzymes, leading to problems that go unnoticed until many years later.

Similarly, what are called *xenobiotics* and *xenoestrogens* — insecticides, vaccinations, antibiotics, and plastics — must also be examined for possible long-term effects on a baby's health and development.

Breast health was influenced while you were developing in your mother. Chemicals that she was exposed to in many cases crossed the placenta and reside inside you even today. Early or chronic exposure of the fetal breast buds to carcinogenic agents can increase the risk of developing breast cancer decades later.

Puberty

Genetics is the major determinant of the timing of puberty, but we know the environment also plays an important role. Studies have shown that girls who live in an area free of toxic substances and are not overweight begin puberty after age fourteen. This is much later than the average American girl, who reaches puberty most often between ages nine and ten. Exposure to hormonal disruptors such as heavy metals, pesticides, petroleum products, antibiotics, and hormonal growth stimulators administered to farm animals plays an integral role in accelerating the growth of breast buds and the uterine lining. Breast health is already being affected since the earlier the onset of puberty, the greater the risk one has of breast cancer in later years.

Once puberty is reached, the ovaries begin to produce sex hormones, resulting in a menstrual cycle. Initially, uterine bleeding can be irregular, because the brain may not send out coordinated signals to the ovaries. However, as the brain's hormonal pathways mature, ovulation ensues and flows become regular and cyclic.

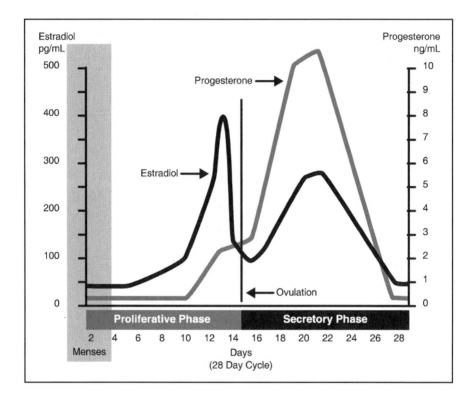

Figure 6. *The twenty-eight-day menstrual cycle.*

The menstrual cycle is divided into two parts:

1. The proliferative, or follicular, phase, which begins on Day One of a normal flow and is dominated by estrogen.

2. The secretory, or luteal, phase, which begins after ovulation and where progesterone and estrogen are present.

During the first part (the proliferative phase) of the more common 28-day cycle, follicular stimulating hormone (FSH) causes the ovaries to produce estrogen over a period of approximately two weeks. This leads to a growth of the uterine lining. Upon reaching a certain level, estrogen causes the brain to secrete luteinizing hormone (LH) that triggers the ovary to release an egg (ovulate).

Ovulation usually occurs around the fourteenth day of the menstrual cycle (where Day One is the first day of good flow) and is the result of a series of finely tuned hormonal events in which the released egg enters the fallopian tube and awaits fertilization.

Following ovulation, the second part of the menstrual cycle, the luteal phase, begins. During this phase the production of progesterone and estrogen together act to stimulate the uterine lining to grow and mature. Progesterone is derived from the empty follicle (known as the *corpus luteum*) that once housed the ovulated egg, and is found in much greater quantities than estrogen. Both hormones must be present in the proper ratio for the uterine lining to accept and nourish the fertilized egg. Progesterone causes maturation and relaxation, whereas estrogen causes growth and stimulation. During this phase, breast cell mitosis (cell replication) is at its greatest level. This explains, in part, the increased incidence of breast tenderness before a menstrual flow. A disturbance in this ratio as manifested by a decline in progesterone can also result in premenstrual syndrome (PMS).

The biologic clock of the *corpus luteum* determines the length of the luteal phase and ceases production of progesterone after approximately fourteen days unless pregnancy intervenes. With the decrease in function of the *corpus luteum*, the uterine lining begins to break down, and menstruation ensues. Most menstrual cycles last twenty-eight days and follow a very regular pattern, while the sloughing of the uterine lining or menstrual flow normally lasts from four to six days. On average, between 30cc and 60cc of blood are lost during a menstrual flow.

> *Note: This is an oversimplification of the twenty-eight-day menstrual cycle, which can vary in length and is dependent upon many factors. A more complex view takes into account other hormones such as insulin, cortisol, and thyroid — hormones that also play important roles, and which will be discussed later.*

Life Phases After the Onset of Puberty

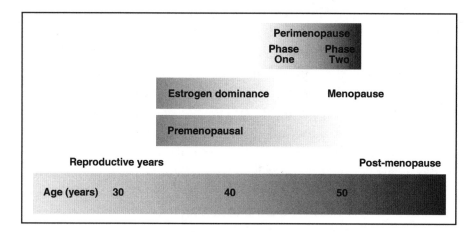

Figure 7. A woman's hormonal transitions.

Reproductive Phase — Menstruation through the Mid-Thirties

For most women, the reproductive years — from around age eighteen to the mid-thirties — are a time of optimal hormonal equilibrium. During the reproductive phase, hormones and health are usually at their best. A young, healthy body can regulate hormones and keep them in remarkable balance.

This phase is when most pregnancies occur. The body is primed for childbearing because there is a sound balance between the endocrine system and the liver-intestine detoxification process. Menstruation is regular and cyclic with the healthiest of eggs being released by the ovaries. The resulting follicle, or *corpus luteum*, produces abundant amounts of progesterone that matures the uterine lining to accept and nourish the fertilized egg — often leading to a successful pregnancy. Still, a woman's body must have a tremendous physiologic reserve and positive lifestyle in order to complete the reproductive phase in optimal health.

Irregular menstrual flows usually result from such conditions as polycystic ovaries or mental and physical stress. Hormonal imbalances can be brought on by genetic predisposition and/or poor living habits, (but rarely because of ovarian aging, as in the Premenopause Phase). In some cases hormonal imbalances due to a stressful environment or unhealthy life choices can lead to symptoms that mimic some aspects of menopause. Chronic stress often causes fatigue, depression, lack of sex drive, and even symptoms of PMS. Inadequate sleep, poor eating habits, and a lack of exercise can also have negative effects.

A diet of fast and processed foods lacks many essential nutrients and can lead to an increased load on the liver-intestinal detoxification system. Pregnancy depletes many of the amino acids that are building blocks for neurotransmitters the brain needs for its optimal function. These deficiencies directly impact not only your mood and energy level but also your hormonal balance. Gestational diabetes, of which excessive weight gain in pregnancy is the major symptom, is linked to an imbalance of insulin (insulin resistance). Women who suffer from this condition have been found to be at risk for breast cancer in later life.

Estrogen-like compounds begin and will continue to accumulate unless dietary changes take place. An overabundance of estrogen can have many detrimental effects. This excess estrogen:

- Stimulates the growth of endometriosis

- Causes excessive cell division and fibrocystic changes in the breast

- Encourages the onset of PMS symptoms including menstrual migraines

- Contributes to heavier menstrual flows

- Increases the incidence of uterine fibroids

A host of other problems can arise during the reproductive phase. For instance, oral contraception (the birth control pill), which is commonly used by women to prevent pregnancy and regulate menses, can also diminish the absorption of certain water-soluble, nutrients, such as vitamin B6 (pyridoxine), that protect against depression.

Irritable bowel disease and even gallbladder problems indicate intestinal absorption problems resulting in even further degradation of the body's detoxification system. Add to this the ingestion of environmental toxins and the rapidly expanding epidemic of obesity in younger and younger women, and the stage is being set for hormonal imbalances now and a real risk for breast disease in the future.

The major disruptive change prior to menopause comes from *estrogen dominance*. Even though estrogen dominance can be present in the reproductive years, it becomes particularly noticeable in your mid- to late thirties.

Premenopause: Mid-Thirties through about Fifty

The premenopause phase is the most tumultuous period in a woman's hormonal history and the most critical phase. During this period hormones fluctuate wildly, sometimes within days or minutes, creating the physical and emotional "roller-coaster" familiar to so many women in early to mid-life.

At this point in your life, it is crucial to have a doctor who understands hormonal balancing. What you and your doctor do in this phase can alleviate many problems, present and future. And properly balancing the hormones in premenopause can determine how you'll experience postmenopause!

The premenopause transition can be subdivided into two periods, each with unique characteristics, treatment, and coping mechanisms:

1. Early premenopause — Estrogen dominance

2. Late premenopause — Perimenopause

For many women, the boundaries between these periods are not always well-defined. Since each individual ages differently, some will not be bothered by the fluctuations in their hormones, while others will be affected with differing degrees of severity.

Early Premenopause: Estrogen Dominance

By the mid- to late thirties, the ovaries have had a reduction in healthy follicles through ovulation and attrition. Hormonal imbalances originate from the aging of ovaries. A woman's ovaries do not suddenly cease to work but over a period of years begin to function in an erratic fashion. This process may begin ten to fifteen years before actual menopause.

The aging of the ovaries (Compartment 2) results in a decreased production of sex hormones. An older egg tends to have a follicle (*corpus luteum*) that produces insufficient amounts of progesterone. The decline in progesterone production precedes that of estrogen and may begin as early as age thirty. Thus estrogen becomes the *dominant* hormone affecting your body. (Estrogen dominance can also be caused by excessive reabsorption and/or inadequate detoxification of estrogen through the liver-intestinal detoxification system.)

Estrogen dominance can begin in adolescence following the onset of ovarian function (menarche) but generally ends, only to appear once again in premenopause.

From a woman's mid- to late thirties through her early forties (the same time estrogen dominance is becoming more pronounced), the body can also be struggling to compensate for emotional stresses, depletion of essential vitamins and minerals, the burden of an overwhelmed liver-intestinal detoxification system, and aging ovaries. This strain is evidenced by a worsening of PMS with symptoms like:

- Mood swings of varying degrees (depression, hostility, irritability, etc.)
- Craving for sweets and chocolate
- Bloating
- Breast tenderness
- Headaches
- Insomnia
- Anxiety
- Fatigue

Further imbalances in Compartments 2 and 3 (the ovaries and non-ovarian endocrine glands) promote these additional symptoms:

- Prolonged, heavy menses
- Weight gain about the midsection of the abdomen
- Fuzzy memory
- Increased disturbances with the gastrointestinal system
- Decreased sex drive
- Hair loss
- Onset of chronic diseases such as arthritis
- Increased allergies

Estrogen dominance can also lead to a thicker uterine lining, bringing on a prolonged heavy flow or flooding and increased fibrocystic changes in the breast (Compartment 4). Benign uterine muscle cell growths, or fibroids, are found with increased frequency. These tumors are estrogen-sensitive and occur in at least fifty percent of women in the premenopause years. Fibroids can cause heavy flows and, if large enough, pelvic discomfort.

> *"I had my white dress on and of course just as I stood up to go to my business meeting, I felt as if the dam had broken. My dress was stained with blood before I made it to the restroom and once again I had no warning."*

Following a pregnancy, some women experience what is known as *shocked ovaries* — the ovary never regains its full function, resulting in inadequate progesterone and even lowered estrogen production. Shocked ovaries seem to be associated with pregnancies that occur later in life (late thirties to early forties).

> *"I am forty-two years old and have had premenopausal symptoms since I gave birth at age thirty-seven. The roller coaster ride is a nightmare and I wonder if there is life at the end of this. I have bleeding that lasts twenty-three to twenty-six days and experience night sweats, hot flashes, insomnia, moodiness, and dizziness. These are about to do me in — especially trying to raise a five-year-old who has lots of energy."*

The aging ovarian follicles not only produce insufficient amounts of progesterone but also decrease the duration of the follicular phase, which can result in a shortening of the menstrual cycle from 28 to 21 days. Ovulation can be delayed or even absent, which leads to irregular flow patterns, and spotting may be noted days before the actual menstrual flow begins.

Late Premenopause: Perimenopause

As the ovary and its follicles continue to age, the hormonal confusion becomes more pronounced. This commonly occurs during the forties and can even continue into the early fifties.

Perimenopause can be divided into two hormonal phases based on the degree of ovarian failure. These are:

1. The frequent, wild fluctuations of estrogen from low to elevated levels, with a continued decline in progesterone.

2. A generalized lowering of estrogen levels with an occasional fluctuation, with little or no progesterone present.

Because the aging body has fewer physiologic reserves to draw on, these hormonal changes can lead to a turbulent transition into menopause. The perimenopause experience can be marked by an increase in the symptoms seen in the early premenopause along with:

- Severe fatigue

- Frequent hot flashes and night sweats that disrupt sleep patterns

- A further loss of cognitive and abstract thought patterns

- Worsening headaches

- Deeper depression

- Unexplained weight gain

- Joint and muscle pain

- Reduction in sex drive

- Vaginal dryness

The transition from one phase to the other may be gradual, but each requires a distinctive treatment approach.

Phase One of Perimenopause

> "I am forty-four years old. My symptoms include erratic periods, mood swings, irritability, fatigue, and hot flashes. I went to my doctor and had a complete physical, Pap smear, and lab work. The nurse called me and told me everything was normal. My husband and mother-in-law say it's the change of life. I wonder if it is possible for my hormone levels to be normal one day and wacky the next? My mother-in-law says that hormone levels change all the time — which is the reason for my mood swings. My symptoms come in spurts that last from several days to two weeks. Then, I might not have them for about a month or so. When I don't have them, I think in my mind, '...Well, maybe I am crazy.' Then all of a sudden, they come back again with my periods being closer together and heavier."

Phase One is characterized by symptoms of both estrogen dominance and estrogen deficiency. The ovaries now begin to receive confusing signals that are derived from the brain's attempt to stabilize estrogen production. Phase One is a combination of too little followed by too much estrogen. Lower estrogen levels reduce the brain's estrogen-sensitive functions such as energy, memory, sleep, moods, and control of the core body temperature.

Initially, the blood level of estrogen rapidly declines. This triggers the release of follicular stimulating hormone (FSH) by the brain in an attempt to wake the ovaries. Erratic spikes of FSH lead to overcompensation by the ovaries, resulting in a temporary elevation of estrogen. This hormonal roller coaster brings on acute physical and neuro-hormonal symptoms that can be very frustrating. With a return to baseline levels, things may get back to normal for a while, but this is only a lull in the storm. At this point, symptoms include occasional night sweats and hot flashes, but the frequency and severity will be more pronounced as you move into Phase Two.

Meanwhile, progesterone is also fluctuating either by being absent because of a lack of ovulation or because of inadequate luteal phase production. Irregular bleeding or intensity, or no bleeding at all for several months followed by flooding, can ensue.

Unexplained weight gain in the mid-abdominal region also can become pronounced. Even though you may exercise and eat the same as in your twenties, the pounds just seem to accumulate. In many cases, lack of exercise and excessive consumption of carbohydrates contribute to this phenomenon. An imbalance of the hormones leptin, insulin, and serotonin may also be instrumental in this mid-life weight gain. Your cells can become insulin-resistant, resulting in carbohydrates being stored as fat instead of being used for energy.

Thyroid and adrenal function also decline in many women, producing symptoms such as cold hands and feet, unexplained hair loss, lack of adequate sleep, susceptibility to infections, and an increase in allergies. In addition, the decline in melatonin and human growth hormone production by the brain can accelerate the aging process.

Blood tests are not always helpful in Phase One because hormonal values fluctuate, sometimes too rapidly to be detected. Low-normal values of estrogen may result in symptoms that disappear when estrogen is raised to a high-normal range. As a result, some women who could clearly benefit from hormone replacement may be denied treatment by practitioners who rely solely on lab values.

Due to misdiagnosis, many women are placed on anti-depressants, sleeping pills, and other pharmaceuticals that may worsen overall health. I believe symptoms should be the guiding factor in whether treatment is appropriate, not the current static blood tests with "one-size-fits-all values."

As perimenopause progresses, production of estrogen and progesterone continues to decrease. At some point, the hormones become almost exhausted and the brain can no longer compensate for the loss. Thus begins the second phase of perimenopause.

Phase Two of Perimenopause (Early Menopause)

> "When I had my first hot flash, I thought I was having intermittent fevers, lasting for 15 to 20 minutes. Mine started in my lower back and moved up to my neck. I just felt a feeling of extreme warmth, no sweating. Over the weeks, it evolved into just intense heat on my neck that spread around to the front of my body. Now, my forehead and nose sweat. Sometimes when they are real intense, my pulse quickens and I get a sick feeling...like the flu. I get weak and shaky and sweat all over. Afterwards, I feel sort of refreshed. Sometimes, I have palpitations...feelings like my heart is beating out of my chest. I can feel my heart beating in my ears and fingertips."

Phase Two is characterized by increasing ovarian resistance to the brain's signals. Estrogen declines to levels that lead to increases in menopause-like symptoms such as hot flashes, night sweats, vaginal dryness, loss of urine, and sporadic uterine bleeding. These symptoms can increase in frequency and severity to the point where they become disruptive.

A sudden drop in estrogen below a certain critical level disrupts the brain's neurocircuits, especially those that control the body's thermostat. This instability results in a hot flash: the sudden reddening of the upper part of the body, accompanied by an intense sensation of heat, and very often, profuse sweating.

In many cases, a lab test will show a modest rise in follicular stimulating hormone (FSH) levels — still below or sometimes consistent with those found in menopause. Estrogen levels tend to be in the low to low-normal range, yet as in Phase One, they may not reflect the severity of the symptoms. Overcompensation by the ovaries with excessive production of estrogen is almost non-existent. Therefore, estrogen-dominant symptoms such as those found in Phase One are no longer present. Since ovulation may have ceased altogether, progesterone is almost entirely absent. It is not uncommon to go several months without a flow.

In Phase Two, symptoms may worsen: more intense and frequent hot flashes and night sweats, the decrease in sex drive, more numerous migraine headaches, anxiety, and depression. Once again, these may be attributed to an overall decrease in ovarian production of estrogen, progesterone, and testosterone. Yet, frequently, women whose lab work indicates their ovaries are no longer functioning (menopausal) still experience uterine bleeding.

Finally, the ovary completely stops producing estrogen and progesterone. Each of the four Reproductive Compartments is affected by this hormonal change, and each will adjust to give rise to the postmenopause life transition.

Late Menopause/Postmenopause

Menopause is thought to occur as a result of the absence of active follicles in the ovaries. Without these follicles, there is a marked decrease in estrogen and progesterone levels, far below that found in women of reproductive age. Eventually, uterine bleeding during perimenopause ceases, and after a period of six to twelve months of no menses, one is said to have been in the menopause.

The average age for menopause in American women is fifty-one, and with current life expectancies, almost 40 percent of a woman's life will be spent in the postmenopause years. (Luckily, humans are unique. Most animal species, including monkeys and chimpanzees, die at the end of their reproductive years.)

> *"I am just now becoming aware of how much menopause is affecting me. It seems everything is falling apart, and I can't count on feeling good from day to day. I'm experiencing all sorts of symptoms, which include waking up in the middle of the night sweating, ongoing aches and pains all over my body, soreness and stiffness in the hips, fatigue almost all of the time, a rapidly expanding belly, weight gain, and aggravation of allergies.*

> *"I have no libido ... and sex sometimes repels me. At my emotional level, it's hell; I frequently have deep, depressive, self-depreciating modes where I am totally internalized or ready to cry at the least little thing. I can't seem to come to terms with my self worth, which right now seems at zero, since I'm not physically or mentally fit to do anything productive.*
>
> *"My memory has been severely affected, and as I reach for a word or a name, I seem to go blank and I can't retrieve it. Sometimes I feel I can't even explain how I feel to my husband, as I can't get to the words. My husband is very compassionate, but this menopausal stuff seems to be beyond understanding. The most alarming effect is the lack of motivation and creative urge. I have nothing to give and nothing inspires me. I have lost my passion, my creativity, and feel dead. It's a scary thing."*

Although the ovaries no longer produce estrogen, they continue to release androgenic hormones such as testosterone. At postmenopause there is a 65 to 70 percent reduction in the body's estrogen production, while androgens may drop 50 to 60 percent. Blood levels of estrogen are not zero because androgens manufactured by the adrenals and the ovaries are being converted to estrogen by fat cells located mainly in the hips, thighs, and abdomen.

The decline in ovarian function also seems connected with the adrenal glands and can lead to both physical and neuro-hormonal imbalances that cause some or all of the following symptoms:

- Night sweats
- Aches and pains
- Soreness and stiffness in the hips
- Fatigue, lack of motivation physically and creatively
- Weight gain/expanding midsection
- Increase in allergies

- Decreased sex drive

- Deep depression

- Oversensitive emotional feelings

- Low self-esteem

- Memory loss

- Vaginal dryness

- Bladder problems

- Insomnia/interrupted sleep

- Heart palpitations

During postmenopause, hormonal production in other glands such as the thyroid and adrenal can decline. With this potential greater reduction in DHEA, thyroid hormone, human growth hormone, pregnenolone, melatonin, and testosterone, the hormonal scene of postmenopause differs from the imbalances of perimenopause. Perimenopause is characterized by the rapid fluctuations of hormone levels over days and hours. In postmenopause, most hormones decline to a steady state. The wild fluctuations come to a halt, along with the frequency and severity of some symptoms. Energy levels are elevated in some (this is referred to as menopausal zest), while others complain of worsening fatigue.

Adaptation to the postmenopause years is related to lifestyle, genetics, and cultural factors. Some women experience severe estrogen withdrawal, while others breeze through relatively unaffected.

Those who experienced PMS in their early to mid-twenties followed by noticeable premenopause difficulties are predisposed to more severe symptoms during postmenopause.

Estrogen replacement plays an integral role during a woman's estrogen-deficient states, which are manifested initially in perimenopause but continue through postmenopause. Confusion concerning the relationship of estrogen and breast cancer has resulted in the needless suffering of many, many women during these transitions. I believe the FEM Centre Breast Care Program can help any woman successfully negotiate these hormonal life transitions because our clinical experience indicates that our program does not result in higher incidences of breast cancer. The earlier in your hormonal transitions that our Breast Care Pyramid is implemented, the greater protection you will have against breast cancer and many other chronic diseases of aging.

CHAPTER 6

The FEM Centre Breast Care Pyramid

Figure 8 shows the FEM Centre Breast Care Pyramid. This pyramid displays the keys to a woman's overall health and is specifically adapted to optimize the health of the breasts. We will explain not only the importance of each section, but how each is intertwined in a wellness plan not only for the breasts but also the brain, heart, and even bones.

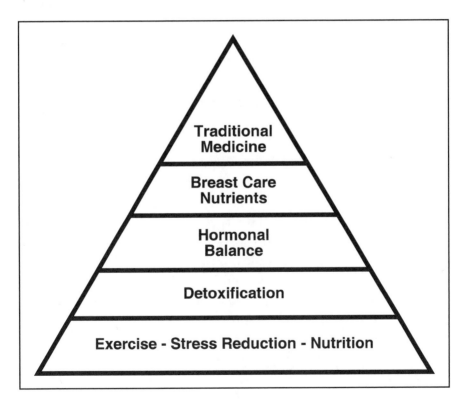

Figure 8. The FEM Centre Breast Care Pyramid.

At the top of the pyramid is *traditional medicine*, which is the most familiar aspect of health and healing. Traditional medicine, as currently practiced, intervenes by treating symptoms once they have appeared. The problem is that traditional medicine does not explicitly emphasize preventing illness and encouraging health. That is why the other components of FEM Centre's Breast Care Pyramid are essential to protect the breast and optimize overall health.

The next section of the pyramid is *breast care nutrients*. Chapter 10 explains how certain vitamins and nutrients can help increase your body's natural defenses, discourage long-term disease, and encourage better health overall. The main purpose of these nutrients is to keep estrogen at a safe level, reducing the negative influence of "bad" estrogens, and promoting the formation of "good" estrogens.

The third section, *hormonal balance,* involves knowing what hormones to balance, and how to assess and adjust their levels. Hormonal balancing is the core of the FEM Centre Breast Care Program and is detailed in Chapter 9.

The fourth section is one of the most important — *detoxification*. During the last few decades, our daily intake of toxins has increased drastically. They are virtually everywhere in our environment: air, water, and food. They come from pesticides, plastics, antibiotics, heavy metals, and the hormones and additives used in our food supply, especially meats. The significance of detoxification and its effect on the rest of the pyramid structure is explained in Chapter 8. Suffice to say, trying to balance your hormones without addressing the toxins in your body is a futile expenditure of time and money.

The base for the pyramid (and the basis for anyone's good health) is *exercise, stress reduction, and nutrition.* These are the most natural medicines you can self-prescribe on a daily basis. They are also inexpensive and readily accessible! Eating the right foods, practicing some form of physical conditioning, and following a lifestyle that avoids stress and toxins creates a solid foundation for optimizing your health. This step of the pyramid is covered in Chapter 7.

CHAPTER 7

Exercise, Stress Reduction, and Nutrition

Exercise — Stress Reduction — Nutrition forms the foundation of the FEM Centre Breast Care Pyramid for one very important reason: Physical conditioning, stress reduction, and proper nourishment are vital for supporting and optimizing the benefits possible with the other parts of the pyramid. The goal of exercise is to increase your body's metabolic rate and halt the loss of muscle; stress reduction helps to detoxify the body and promotes the balancing of hormones; and good nutrition aids in keeping the body cleansed while strengthening its immune system defenses.

Exercise

Aerobic exercise is one form of physical activity that appears to halt both weight gain and aging. In addition, aerobic exercise helps strengthen your heart and lungs. Aerobic exercise produces an oxygen-driven metabolic state, which allows the body to selectively incorporate fat as the main source of fuel. As a result, you begin to enter a fat-burning zone with a subsequent decrease in body fat percentage. This type of exercise is characterized by any moderate, continuous physical activity that creates a greater demand for oxygen in the body. Think of it as long, slow, distance training. Training in this fat burning zone should feel relaxed and light. Examples would include walking, cycling, jogging, swimming, and aerobic dance, just to name a few. This is not the same exercise as one gets with tennis, sprinting, or sports that require short, intense bursts of physical activity. If you want to burn excess body fat, aerobic exercise is the answer.

Don't worry if you are not exercising enough. One of the easiest ways to get started with aerobic exercising is walking. Studies show that, for many people, walking burns almost as many calories as seemingly more rigorous exercises like jogging, swimming, or aerobic classes. Walking is a weight-bearing activity that helps to maintain bone and prevent osteoporosis. Walking doesn't require any special training or equipment skills. Just get a pair of comfortable, cushioned shoes. It is convenient and easy to fit into almost any schedule. The intensity of walking can be easily varied according to the physical condition and needs of the individual. Ultimately, you should strive to walk briskly from 30 to 40 minutes at a time for a distance of two miles, four times a week.

When we look at someone's exercise plan, frequently it falls short of the exercise intensity required to be in the fat-burning zone. Heart-rate monitoring is an excellent way to measure your exercise intensity and endurance. Your heart rate is an important barometer that can be used to gauge not only your fitness but also the quality of a workout session. Think of it as an efficiency rating for your entire body. Monitoring your heart rate during exercise allows you to judge the fat-burning efficiency of your activity while also preventing overexertion.

As you become more comfortable with a program such as walking, we suggest that you obtain an exercise heart rate monitor. Using the data supplied by the monitor and depending on the medicines that you are taking, the safe heart rate range needed to reach the fat-burning zone can then be calculated by your physician.

Resistance (or strength) training is the second type of exercise. Whereas aerobic or endurance activities are designed for losing fat and maintaining cardiopulmonary fitness, resistance training is designed to increase strength and flexibility.

The loss of muscle mass through the aging process can be reversed with this type of exercise. Muscles are extremely important for weight control since they consume 50 to 90 percent of all the calories burned daily. Bones also benefit from strength training, which can reverse the process of osteoporosis. We suggest that your strength training emphasize those muscle groups and movements that are important in daily activities. Below we list a basic weight-training schedule. You might consider consulting an exercise professional or personal trainer before starting.

Resistance Training

In the following section we describe a series of individual exercises using a fitness ball, lunges, and resistance bands that when combined form a "whole body" exercise routine. If you are new to resistance training, begin by completing just one set of 12 to 17 repetitions once a week of each of the seven exercises. As you get stronger consider two, then three sets of 8 to 12 repetitions two to three times per week. *Note: It is very important to allow a day of rest before working the same muscle group again.*

The body burns the majority of fat not during the actual exercise but in repairing the muscles afterwards. Therefore, you need to break down the muscles during each exercise period. You can tell this is happening when you begin to feel fatigued three-fourths of the way through a set. If you are not noticing this fatigue, you need to increase the resistance or repetitions.

Ball wall squats — primary focus: quadriceps

Exercise: Stand, leaning against ball in small of your back, against wall. Place feet hip-width apart, toes turned outward slightly with knees bent. Descend to a right angle, as if sitting in an invisible chair in a "down–2–3–pause, up–2–3" count for 12 to 17 repetitions per set initially. As your initial program becomes less challenging, increase resistance by adding additional sets of repetitions and/or add small free weights in each hand.

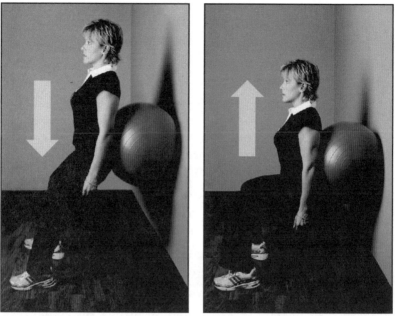

Down–2–3–pause   Up–2–3

Breathing: Inhale on way to seated position. Exhale on way back up to slightly bent knees.

To increase resistance: Slow down and increase duration of pause in seated position to 1 to 3 seconds. Hold free weights in hands.

Ball ham curls — primary focus: hamstrings

Exercise: Lie on back on carpet or mat. Place heels and part of calves on ball. Roll ball back toward your buttocks in a "back–2–3" count until the soles of your feet are flat on ball. Return to starting position by extending legs, in a "out–2–3" count, rolling ball out and away from you. Complete 12 to 17 repetitions per set initially. As your program becomes less challenging, add additional sets of repetitions.

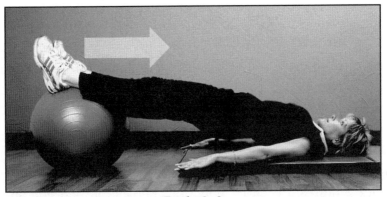

Back–2–3

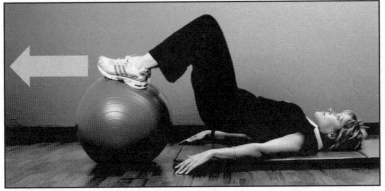

Out–2–3

Breathing: Exhale as you roll ball back, and inhale as you extend to starting position.

To increase resistance: Slow down and/or change hands from palms down to palms up.

Stationary lunges — primary focus: quadriceps (front of thighs)

Note: In this exercise, the front leg is the "working" leg and your center of gravity should be such that most of your weight is on the heel of your front foot. This is a "compound" exercise so it also utilizes hamstrings and glutes as well!

<u>Exercise:</u> Stand with left leg forward, bent slightly and right leg behind, bent slightly, balancing on toe, with feet shoulder-width apart. Use chair only if you need it for balance and with light fingertips only. Chest up, abs in.

Tip: Curl toe upward in shoe of front foot to force weight onto heel and keep you from allowing knee to go over toe (which is stressful on knee). You should have very little weight on back leg.

Bend both legs in right angle as you move in downward motion in a "down–2–3, up–2–3" count. Repeat with right leg forward, left leg back. Complete 12 to 17 repetitions per set on each side initially. As your program becomes less challenging, add additional sets of repetitions.

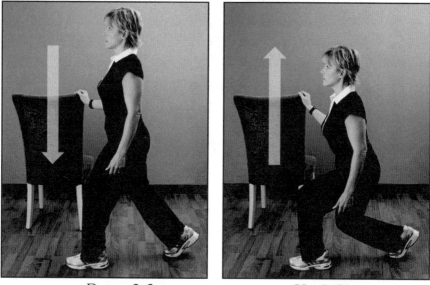

Down–2–3   Up–2–3

<u>Breathing:</u> Inhale on way down to mid-point, and exhale upward to return without ever fully straightening legs.

<u>To increase resistance:</u> Slow down and/or hold free weights in each hand.

Sitting latissimus row — primary focus: latissimus dorsi (back)

Exercise: Sit with legs fully extended in front or slightly bent. Chest is up and abs are in. Wrap "medium" resistance band around feet twice, holding handgrips in each hand with palms facing inward. Relax or drop shoulders down and squeeze shoulder blades together before moving both elbows back as if strings are pulling them back in a "back–2–3–pause, forward–2–3" count. Complete 12 to 17 repetitions per set initially. As your program becomes less challenging, add additional sets of repetitions.

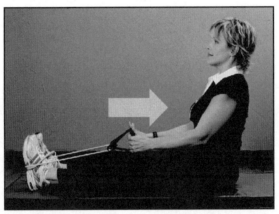

Back–2–3–pause

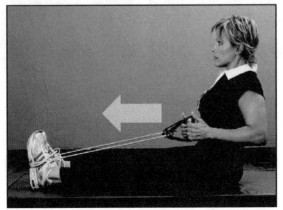

Forward–2–3

Breathing: Exhale as you go back, and inhale as you return to starting position, never fully extending arms to straight.

To increase resistance: Slow down or increase resistance level of band.

Seated tricep extension — primary focus: triceps (back of upper arm)

Exercise: Sit, leaning forward on front half of chair seat with medium-resistance band wrapped around back of chair. Remember, chest up, abs in. Start with arms shoulder-width apart, elbows bent at a right angle, at chin level. Straighten both arms to full extension in a "1–2–3–reach, back–2–3" count for 12 to 17 repetitions per set initially. As your program becomes less challenging, add additional sets of repetitions.

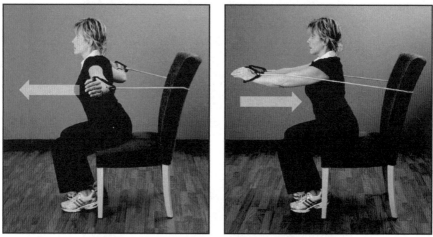

1–2–3–reach   back–2–3

Breathing: Exhale during extension, and inhale upon return.

To increase resistance: First slow down. Second, increase to next band resistance level.

Bicep band curls — primary focus: biceps (front of upper arm)

Note: In the following two exercises the "ready position" is standing with feet hip-width apart, knees bent, and buttocks out.

Exercise: Stand in ready position with feet hip-width apart on band with handgrips in each hand, palms open and up. Start with elbows slightly bent, lifting palms up toward chest. Pause at chest level for one count and descend to starting position in an "up 2–3–pause; down–2–3–pause" count for 12 to 17 repetitions per set initially. As your program becomes less challenging, add additional sets of repetitions.

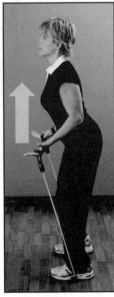 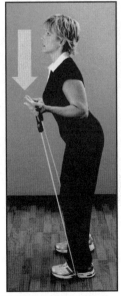

Up 2–3–pause   Down–2–3–pause

Breathing: Exhale during upward motion, and inhale as you lower hands.

To increase resistance: First, slow down. Second, move feet outward for a wider stance and three, increase to next band resistance level.

Standing lateral raises — primary focus: deltoids (shoulders)

Exercise: Stand in ready position with one foot forward, standing on "light" resistance band. Start with hands at sides, then lift-up with back of hands toward the ceiling. Never go higher than the plane of your shoulders. Pause and return to starting positions in an "up–2–3–pause, down–2–3" count for 12 to 17 repetitions per set initially. As your program becomes less challenging, add additional sets of repetitions.

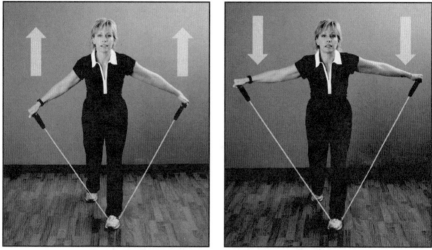

Up–2–3–pause   Down–2–3

Breathing: Exhale as you bring band up, and inhale as you descend, never letting tension off band.

To increase resistance: First slow down. Second, stand on resistance band with feet side-by-side on band, widening your stance over time as repetitions become easier. Third increase to next band resistance level.

Daily Breast Massage and Chest Exercise

Centuries ago, Taoist healers used breast massage to promote breast health. Today, this lymphatic breast massage has been reintroduced to help the breasts dispose of potentially carcinogenic substances.

The body uses the lymph system to remove toxins that can accumulate in breast tissue. Exercise, breast-feeding, and massage act to enhance the function of this system by stimulating the breast. We have frequently documented dramatic improvement in thermographic images of the breast by simply using lymphatic breast massage.

Breast-feeding with its ensuing nipple stimulation leads to the release of oxytocin. The resulting contraction of muscle fibers in the breast improves circulation in the lymph system. In fact, women who have breast-fed their offspring in excess of 20 months experience a 50 percent decrease in their incidence of breast cancer.

Breast massage/stimulation can be undertaken alone or with the assistance of a partner.

Taoist Breast Massage

- Rub your palms together until they feel warm

- Cup your palms over your breasts

- Gently rub in a circular, outward motion away from the cleavage and toward the armpits; you are trying to move the breasts away from each other, not squeeze them together

- Taoist healers recommend performing 36 circles

Breast Massage

- Lie face-up on a flat surface

- Extend your left arm over your head

- With the fingers of the right hand, squeeze and/or gently rub the left nipple for a few minutes, using only the amount of pressure that feels comfortable

- Grasp the lower portion of the breast, squeeze, and release in a pumping motion. Move upward and outward. This entire sequence should last three minutes.

- Repeat the above actions on the right breast

You can also perform breast massage using progesterone cream, vitamin E oil, or evening primrose oil. Some women's breasts may be too sore or sensitive for massage, indicating a progesterone deficiency or an excessive estrogen level. Implementing our breast care program is likely to diminish breast tenderness and fibrocystic changes.

Exercise is also helpful in quickening the circulation of the breasts' lymph system, resulting in an overall tissue cleansing. Studies in Denmark show that women who never wear bras have a much lower incidence of breast cancer, which indicates that wearing a tight-fitting bra can inhibit the breasts' lymph circulation.

The *Pectoral Squeeze* is a superb exercise that develops and strengthens your chest wall muscles (pecs). These muscles are your natural support, a muscular "wonder bra." This exercise can be used in conjunction with either of the breast massage techniques described above.

The Pectoral Squeeze

- Stand in front of a mirror to observe how the pectoral muscles work to lift the breasts

- Extend your arms in front at shoulder height

- Bend your arms at the elbows until the forearms are at a 90-degree angle

- Tighten your hands into fists; don't let the elbows droop

- Spread the bent arms to the side and begin to bring them in front so that both elbows almost touch — in and out, in and out

- Do this about 20 times a day

As stated in a women's newsletter, "It's obvious that breasts were made to be touched, gently squeezed, and otherwise pleasantly stimulated." Science has confirmed this remark.

Stress Reduction

Eastern medicine, as well as our own Native American medicine, realized the importance of the mind-body connection in one's overall health. These ancient forms of healing consider that certain illnesses in the physical body often result from imbalances in the mind or spiritual realm.

A common problem that arises in modern society is the hectic, stressful lifestyles that many of us have become accustomed to. The word "stress" is heard all too often. In order to complete the whole picture for optimal health and well-being, you should consider taking time out during a busy day for stress reduction.

Stress has the potential to adversely affect every organ system in your body. Disruption of harmony between mind and body may result from lack of sleep, overwork, monetary difficulties, and unre-solved issues that are common in our complex Western society.

Women have expanded their role to provide extra, if not sole, in-come for the family. Not only do they become responsible for taking care of the family in a traditional sense, but now they must also compete in the demanding world of business. This added responsi-bility creates stressful conflicts.

Chronic stress results in the release of the hormones adrenaline and cortisol from the adrenal glands. Adrenaline acts to block for-mation of healthy hormones, while cortisol increases insulin levels, which in turn leads to the production of destructive agents.

An increase in adrenaline can lead to elevated blood pressure, and cortisol breaks down substances in the body instead of building and replenishing. Overeating and lack of sleep frequently result from stress. You begin to add extra weight while becoming run-down. Over time, your immune system can be affected.

The detrimental effects of stress on the breast should not be ig-nored. On numerous occasions I have consulted with women, who after experiencing a traumatic emotional event in the recent past such as divorce, were suddenly diagnosed with breast cancer.

Good health (including that of the breast) and weight manage-ment involve more than just eating better, correcting hormonal im-balances, and exercising. Your body needs appropriate amounts of rest and relaxation for optimal physical and mental health.

Here are some tips:

- Start by performing deep breathing for five minutes once a day. This provides a link between the conscious and unconscious. As you turn attention to breathing, you will begin to relax and enter a state of meditation. Extend your breathing practices to several times throughout the day.

- Begin daily stretching for at least five minutes at any convenient time. Yoga and Pilates offer formal systems of stretching the body.

- When you become trapped in a "hurry mode" all the time, learn to pause and take a few deep breaths.

- Exercise can be a *natural* form of relaxation and mood elevation. Take a walk in a park or a botanical garden area that provides a pleasant visual experience. Exercise with a friend if possible.

- Begin to take a "news fast" at least one to two days a week. Emotional ups and downs frequently result from the state of the world as reported in the news. Studies have shown that people who watch, listen to, and/or read a lot of news have a more negative view of the world at large, and they often overestimate the current level of crime in their area compared with actual data. Try to avoid reading or listening to the news and you'll notice that your attitude toward the world quickly becomes more positive. This allows you an emotional break from constant turmoil.

- Listen to music that you find particularly relaxing. Reading is another excellent means of escape and pleasure. Hobbies can also be very rewarding.

- Improve the quality of your sleep. Try to establish and maintain as regular a pattern of nightly sleep as possible. And before going to bed, begin to wind down your activities and relax.

- Spirituality, whether through religion or meditation, offers one the ability to place things in proper perspective and deal with external turmoil.

- When the world "pulls your strings," realize that your mind wields a mighty pair of scissors.

Toxic thoughts generate toxic molecules. Happy thoughts make happy molecules. Therefore, and not surprisingly, women who have breast cancer along with a positive attitude or outlook have an almost 50 percent increase in their survival rate.

Nutrition — The FEM Centre Nutrition Plan

Good nutrition provides your body with sources of energy, cellular building blocks, and stimulus for hormone action. Little wonder that breast health is so dependent upon food intake.

All of us, at one time or another, have required prescriptions or have purchased over-the-counter medications to alleviate various ailments. To many this practice has become so routine that one is left to wonder how anyone can survive without a well-stocked medicine cabinet. Even worse, the reliance on pharmaceuticals has become a mass-media mantra further contributing to the all-too-common perception that growing older will inevitably require taking multiple medications.

What did people use before the development of our technically advanced medical system and its abundant array of sophisticated drugs? How was our species able to survive and flourish? And, what do people in less developed countries do for headaches, heartburn, depression, or joint and muscle aches?

There is one simple answer that is frequently overlooked — a unique and powerful medicine, created by nature, and designed especially for us — food. *You are what you eat* is more than a cliché; it's a basic truism that has been known for centuries.

Our breast care program endorses and relies on the concept that food should be your first medicine of choice — a paradigm quite different from that of traditional medicine. We suggest you forget the medicine cabinet and instead use the suggestions in this chapter to stock your refrigerator and pantry. Preventing the chronic diseases of aging, especially our current breast cancer epidemic, begins with proper nutrition.

Your body requires a constant stream of information that is translated by your genes into the instructions that govern cellular functions. Good information leads to healthy cellular activity and overall wellness of the body. Poor food choices can send the wrong signals, resulting in poor health.

During the last fifty years, our diet has changed dramatically. With the appearance of microwave ovens, fast-food restaurants, and hundreds of chemical additives and preservatives, Americans have become well-fed and undernourished. The state of our national health has mirrored this change, as evidenced by dramatic increases in the chronic diseases of aging occurring in ever-younger age groups.

The last few decades have seen an astonishing increase in obesity among Americans. More than 50 percent of the population is now considered overweight. While some of this can be attributed to our leading a more sedentary lifestyle than prior generations that spent much of their lives performing labor-intensive tasks, there is also a direct correlation between weight problems and the development and subsequent infiltration of processed foods into the American diet. In the case of breast cancer, the adverse effects of obesity are clearly illustrated — excessive weight increases one's risk by 1.8 to almost 2.99 times. This even exceeds the risk associated with the use of Prempro.

Our Prehistoric Legacy

Our genetic makeup is a product of many thousands of years of selective development. Throughout this period of development a very specific diet has allowed the human species to survive and multiply. Yet, in the span of a few decades that diet has been significantly altered. Even though twenty or thirty years is but a blink of an eye in our long biological history, this radical change in diet has caused a shock to the system, resulting in an extraordinary gain in body weight and other equally disturbing health problems that contemporary humans are experiencing.

For thousands of generations, humans existed as hunter-gatherers. Their diet consisted of water, fruits, vegetables, nuts, and the lean meat of wild game. There were no grain or dairy products in the prehistoric diet, and needless to say, the human digestive system did not come into contact with pesticides, chemical additives, preservatives, and other recent scientific "marvels." (Two major contributors to contemporary health problems, alcohol and tobacco, were as yet unknown.) On the whole, the environments and diets of our ancestors were sufficiently clean, balanced, and nutritious to sustain and nurture the species.

So, how did these people fare? As late as the 1970s, scientists were able to study indigenous people with prehistoric diets as described above. In general, deficiencies of such nutrients as folic acid and vitamin B12 did not exist, and few women suffered from a lack of iron, even during pregnancy and breast-feeding. It was common to find many people who lived into their late seventies or eighties. Due to lower body fat and the absence of dietary xenoestrogens, women had an average onset of menstruation at fifteen and a half years of age, well above the current average among American females. But, most astonishing of all of the observations — blood pressure did not seem to increase with age, the elderly were rarely affected with degenerative diseases, and breast cancer was essentially non-existent.

More Recent Changes

Around 10,000 to 11,000 years ago, the modern human species *Homo sapiens* began to settle into agricultural villages. Women abandoned foraging and became more sedentary. Grain was cultivated and harvested, and livestock was raised and slaughtered for villagers' consumption. Certain tribes in modern-day Africa serve as present-day equivalents to these humans and show that this lifestyle change gives rise to an increase in overall body weight, an earlier onset of puberty, and a host of new degenerative diseases.

It should be no surprise, then, that we see these same penalties affecting our own population. Take this agricultural diet and add to it the overly processed, chemical-laden foods of the "modern" diet and the toxic environment created by technological "progress" and you have a prescription for disaster — uncontrolled increases in body weight and degenerative diseases, both occurring in ever-younger age groups.

We are faced with a problem of epic proportions — primeval genes having to cope with strange new environmental and nutritional variables for which they were never designed.

Solutions

Your inherited genetic information combined with your lifestyle makes your metabolism as unique as your fingerprints. This means your path to better breast and body health is both complex and individualized. There can be no one-diet-fits-all solution because your body has individualized metabolic needs requiring its own unique quantities and types of food. This is why our plan focuses on nutrition as opposed to diet.

As we age, our genes switch from metabolizing and burning calories to storing and hoarding calories. This most often leads to the ever-increasing girth of our midsection, among other places, when we pass from youth to middle age. In order to mitigate our genes' tendency to gear our metabolism to that of a hibernating polar bear, we must avoid fad diets and magic pills and instead follow a comprehensive, principle-based method of food consumption.

It is my belief that proper nutrition encourages not only weight control but also diminishes the risk of acquiring breast cancer.

The Five Dietary Principles to Promote Breast Health

The dietary principles that allow us to realize our goals of weight control, breast health, and longevity are:

1. Eat a predominantly plant-based diet with approximately 30 percent of your daily caloric input derived from protein. Avoid processed foods.

2. Maintain a proper balance of fats and oils.

3. Reduce or eliminate salt, food additives, caffeine, and coloring agents.

4. Drink six to eight glasses of purified water and/or other healthy beverages daily.

5. Determine and adhere to the number of calories needed to maintain an optimal body weight.

1. Eat your vegetables (Mother was right) — and your protein

Fresh fruits and vegetables are the most effective and least expensive "natural" medicines available today for optimizing your health. A predominantly plant-based diet high in fiber, essential fatty acids, antioxidants, and phytochemicals has been shown to decrease the risk of cancer, heart disease, strokes, and other chronic illnesses.

Positive anti-aging and anti-breast cancer results can be derived from the following:

- Carotenes — found in green leafy vegetables, and yellow- and orange-colored fruits and vegetables

- Glucosinolates — found in broccoli, Brussels sprouts, cabbage, and cauliflower

- Non-vitamin A active pigments — found in red and purple fruits and vegetables

- Flavonoids — found in abundance in citrus, berries, onions, parsley, legumes, and green tea

Balancing Basics

Three critical components of nutrition are carbohydrates, protein, and fat. These elements are essential to a healthy diet, but what is also important is their relationship to one another. To address this, the FEM Centre Breast Care Program recommends the following ratio to guide your daily diet:

- Carbohydrates — 40 to 50 percent of calories

- Proteins — 30 percent of calories

- Fats — 20 to 30 percent of calories

Other important considerations include fiber (the FEM Centre recommends at least 25 to 35 grams per day), and knowing the appropriate types of carbohydrates, proteins, and fats to ingest in order to achieve the greatest benefit.

Complex Carbohydrates

There are two basic types of carbohydrates: simple and complex. Simple carbohydrates consist of one, two, or at most three molecules of sugar attached together. Complex carbohydrates are made up of hundreds to thousands of sugar links. The complex carbs are further divided into high fiber and low fiber. High fiber complex carbs exhibit the greatest health benefits.

Carbohydrates directly impact your blood sugar levels. A steady blood sugar level minimizes mood swings, encourages mental focus, stimulates fat burning, and increases energy, strength, endurance, and metabolism — whereas dramatic fluctuations in your blood sugar level can lead to dizziness, drowsiness, fatigue, restlessness, and/or irritability. You have probably experienced these symptoms after a big lunch of the wrong foods (simple or low-fiber complex carbs). This mid-afternoon malaise can easily be avoided by eating the proper foods at the proper time.

Carbohydrates also perform another important function: They assist the brain in absorbing tryptophan and other substances needed for sleep. Tryptophan is converted into serotonin and finally melatonin, which is a powerful nighttime hormone.

High-fiber complex carbs are included in the lower glycemic food groups, which means they have the least effect on blood sugar levels.

In tune with your circadian rhythms, you should eat a larger portion of healthy, low-glycemic/high-fiber complex carbohydrates (see Appendix D) along with an adequate, but smaller amount, of protein at night. By enhancing your ability to sleep, you can stabilize your moods and balance your body's hormone production.

Note: In Chapter 10, I listed a limited number of antioxidant supplements that should be included in a daily multivitamin. This list is dwarfed by what is available in whole foods such as fruits and vegetables. For example, an apple contains more than nine hundred substances that not only have antioxidant-like effects but are more effectively absorbed by your intestines. It should not be surprising that regular consumption of apples has already been shown to prevent breast tumors in animals. "Several apples a day could keep breast cancer away."

High-fiber-containing complex carbohydrates are recommended because of their ability to stabilize insulin levels. The following items should be included in your nutrition plan:

Vegetables

Non-starchy vegetables are an excellent complex-carbohydrate source of natural fiber, vitamins, and minerals when prepared properly and stored knowledgeably.

It is recommended that you consume no less than five servings daily (a serving equals one cup) with at least two servings at both lunch and dinner.

Most commonly served in the United States are:

Asparagus	Jalapenos	Swiss chard
Bell peppers	Kale	Raw tomatoes
Broccoli	Lettuce (dark, leafy)	Turnip greens
Brussels sprouts	Mushrooms	Watercress
Cabbage	Mustard greens	
Raw carrots	Onions	
Cauliflower	Parsley	
Celery	Peppers (red, yellow)	
Collard greens	Radishes	
Cucumbers	Snap peas	
Dandelion greens	Snow peas	
Eggplant	Shallots	
Garlic	Spinach	
Ginger root	Spaghetti squash	
Green beans	Summer squash	

Minimize your intake of starchy vegetables. Although they contain fiber, they can be a problem for people with candida.

Acorn squash	Leeks
Artichokes	Lima beans
Beets	Okra
Butternut squash	Potatoes
Cooked carrots	Pumpkin
Corn	Sweet potatoes
Green peas	Turnips

Vegetables should be at least 60 percent of your diet if you are following our guidelines for optimal digestion and acid/alkaline balance. I recommend they be consumed raw, or prepared as follows: steamed, sautéed, roasted, cooked in soups, or in vegetable pâtés.

A healthy salad should be a daily addition to your diet since it is a quick and fresh source of dark, leafy greens.

Fruits

Fruits are complex carbohydrates in their whole form because they contain fiber. However, since they are high in simple sugars, we rate them according to the Glycemic Index (Appendix D).

Portion sizes need to reflect each individual's current metabolism and activity level. As a general rule one should consume only two servings of fruits daily.

Candida sufferers who have significant symptoms including itching, brain fog, digestive gas, and bloating should avoid all fruits (with the exception of Granny Smith apples, berries, lemons, and limes) until detoxification is complete (see Chapter 8).

Fruits are best consumed alone or with protein fats such as yogurt and kefir.

Lowest Glycemic Index fruits (with recommended serving size):

Blackberries	¾ cup
Blueberries	¾ cup
Boysenberries	¾ cup
Grapefruit	½ medium
Raspberries	1 cup
Strawberries	1 cup
Kiwi	1 large
Avocados	1 small

Mid-Glycemic Index fruits (with recommended serving size):

Apples	1 small
Apricots	3 medium
Cantaloupe	1¼ cup
Cherries	12
Honeydew	⅛ medium
Mango	½ small
Nectarine	1 small
Orange	1 small
Papaya	1 cup
Peach	1 medium
Pear	½ large
Pineapple	¾ cup
Plums	2 medium
Pomegranate	½ fruit

Highest Glycemic Index fruits (with recommended serving size):

Banana	½ small
Dates	2 medium
Figs	2 medium
Grapes	15 small
Prunes	3 medium
Raisins	2 tablespoons
Watermelon	1¼ cup

Grains

Note: There is no requirement for grains in our diet, and many people have suffered greatly from food allergies related to grain consumption and molds that live on poorly stored grains. Yet, proper selection of "whole grains" has been shown time and time again to be protective against cancer, heart disease, diabetes, and excessive weight gain. Whole grains, which we have listed below, are excellent sources of dietary fiber, nourish the digestive tract and are loaded with antioxidants.

Allowed in 15-gram increments per serving (up to three servings daily):

- Organic brown rice
- Organic wild rice
- Organic quinoa
- Organic amaranth
- Organic millet
- Organic buckwheat
- Organic popcorn (once-a-week treat)
- Organic blue corn tortillas
- Yellow corn tortillas (dining out)

You should eat as little refined flour, crackers, chips, cereals, desserts, or snacks as possible. I suggest, when shopping for groceries, you avoid purchasing items that contain white flour or sugar. If these items are readily available, you will eventually succumb to the temptation to eat them. When eating at a restaurant, politely ask the waiter not to place bread on the table. This will remove the temptation to indulge before the main course is served.

Protein

The benefits of protein for body function and tissue repair are considerable. It is the primary source of essential amino acids for building lean muscle mass. Proteins from lean, clean sources boost hormonal and immune system function. They provide the building blocks of neurotransmitters that govern mood and many other hormonal functions. The various protein sources contain few if any carbohydrates, so they are an ideal aid for diabetics who must stabilize their blood sugar and dieters who must lose weight to regain their health.

Due to protein's acidic nature, excessive consumption of animal protein and meats high in saturated fat may result in a loss of bone mass or inflammation of body tissues in certain individuals. Lamb, beef, chicken, goat, etc., should be eaten with fresh herbs like ginger, fennel, garlic, wheat-free soy sauce, or dark green leafy vegetables. People with chronic digestive complaints may have insufficient levels of the digestive enzymes (pancreatin, lipase, and hydrochloric acid) needed to break down animal foods well. Also, be aware that growth hormones, antibiotics, and elevated levels of toxic chemicals are regularly found in commercial livestock. Leave room for digestion and chew your meat thoroughly and thoughtfully. Candida sufferers should avoid aged and smoked meats.

Be careful to cook meats just until they are done. Do not overcook them or char them using an open flame.

Our recommendation is that sedentary adults eat no more than three ounces of meat or poultry per serving.

Animal-based Proteins to Avoid

- Pork bacon, ham, hotdogs
- Commercial lunchmeat with nitrates
- Canned meats
- Heavy-fat cuts such as brisket, liver, rib steaks
- Fast-food hamburgers

Animal–based Proteins to Enjoy

Poultry — Serving size: 3 to 6 ounces; eat three to four times weekly

- Free-range organic chicken (white meat only)
- Organic turkey (white meat only)

Fish — Serving size: 3 to 4 ounces; eat up to three times weekly. Mercury contamination is a concern so be aware of the source, especially for albacore tuna, shark, swordfish, king mackerel, and tilefish.

- Mahi-Mahi
- Tilapia
- Trout
- Flounder
- Lowest in saturated fats:
  - Haddock
  - Cod
  - Scallops
- Highest in omega-3 fatty acids:
  - Salmon (Wild Alaskan or Copper River)
  - Sardines

Red Meat — Serving size: 3 ounces; eat three times a week or less

- Grass-fed sirloin and select cuts for leanness ("round" cuts)
- Lamb shank, chops
- Buffalo
- Venison
- Ostrich
- Emu

Dairy —

- Free-range eggs, two to four daily is permissible
- Full-fat Kefir cheese, 2 to 3 ounces daily, or liquid Kefir, up to ½ cup daily
- Full-fat yogurt (plain, organic)
- Cheeses*: feta, goat cheese — preferably organic; mozzarella, ricotta, string cheese are well-tolerated if no allergy to casein or lactose exists
- Fresh organic butter and ghee — serving size 1 tablespoon

*Avoid if you suffer from fibroids or respiratory disorders.

Note: Dietary fats should not exceed 20 to 30 percent of the diet. Be sure to count all sources such as dairy products, medicinal oils, nuts, and seeds.

Vegetarian Proteins — Serving size: ½ cup or less; eat seven times a week

Vegetarian proteins contain complex carbohydrates and fiber, and are good sources of vitamins and minerals. However, be careful that you do not exceed your glycemic load (see Appendix D).

- Soy foods
  - Tempeh
  - Natto
  - Miso
  - Tofu curd
  - Edamame (fresh)
  - Black soybeans (lowest in carbohydrates)
  - Regular soybeans
- Legumes (beans)
  - Lentils
  - Aduki
  - Split peas
  - Pinto/ refried
  - Falafel
  - Hummus (lowest in carbohydrates)
  - Fava
  - Navy
  - Broad
  - White
  - Blackeyed peas

Notes: People who have problems with digestion may require high-quality enzymes to help break down legumes. Soaking lessens cooking time and improves digestion. Sprouted legumes are highly recommended. Candida sufferers should avoid beans until digestion allows.

The FEM Centre nutrition plan is an excellent way to prevent the growth of fungi in our bodies. This is particularly important since their toxins (mycotoxins) have been shown to be cancer-causing Some have even gone so far as to suggest that many cancers including breast have a fungal etiology. Both can exist in a low oxygen environment, prefer sugar as their energy source, invade and destroy surrounding tissue, and are eradicated by similar medications such as ketoconazole (Nizoral), anastrozole (Arimidex), and letrozole (Femara). It would seem that a diet hostile to the growth of fungi would also be hostile to breast cancer.

Daily Action Items

- At least four to five servings of vegetables
- Two servings of fresh fruit. Avoid foods with a high glycemic index (see Appendix D)
- 25 to 35 grams of fiber
- 4 to 6 ounces of protein (free-range, skinless poultry, or legumes with some fish)
- One to three servings of whole grain (preferably brown or basami rice) allowed but not required

Note: Fresh, organic, vine-ripened fruits and vegetables are preferred when available. In order to preserve inherent enzymes, they should be eaten raw or lightly steamed.

2. Maintain a Proper Balance of Fats/Oils

I suggest you forget about the public image of fat as being bad for you. Instead focus on the fact that in spite of all the hype about removing fat from our food (with low-fat cookies, chips, and ice creams), we have still seen a dramatic increase in obesity. It is important to understand that some fats are good for the breast and should be included in your diet, while others should be avoided or at least minimized. It is the amount and type of fat contained in your diet that affects the breast.

Fats are created from fatty acids and form the building blocks for powerful hormones called eicosanoids. These hormones influence virtually every structure in your body, including the immune system, the brain, breasts, ovaries, and heart. Fats also supply the raw materials needed to make cell membranes. This skin-like structure is a cell's interface with the outside environment, controlling what comes into and out of the cell.

We need certain types of fat in our diet in order to survive and remain healthy. Healthy dietary fats should account for 20 to 30 percent of your daily caloric intake. One of the most important recent discoveries is that eating a balanced ratio of essential fatty acids is necessary for good health.

Unfortunately, the typical American diet is loaded with the type of fats that are dangerous and harmful to your body. At the same time, the American diet is deficient in those fats that contribute to fitness and vitality. To make matters worse, many diet plans are mistakenly based on a low-fat, high-carbohydrate meal, which only increases weight problems. We consume too many simple carbohydrates, which not only cause our population to grow fatter, but also contribute to an increase in breast cancer and degenerative illnesses such as diabetes, Alzheimer's, and heart disease.

For these reasons, our breast care program urges you to avoid a low-fat, high-carbohydrate diet.

Fats can be divided into three categories:

- **Saturated fats:** These fats contain no double chemical bonds between carbon atoms and are completely saturated with hydrogen atoms. Saturated fats are found mainly in dairy products, meat, and animal fats. You can easily recognize these fats since they are solid at room temperature rather than liquid. Studies show that women who have diets high in saturated fats are at greater risk for breast cancer.

- **Monosaturated fats:** *Mono* is Greek for "one." There is one double bond that connects two of the carbons in this fat. This reduces the number of hydrogen atoms, compared with saturated fats. Olive oil, peanut oil, avocados, canola oil, and most nuts are high in monosaturated fats, which are considered healthy fats. The Mediterranean diet, which has been associated with lower breast cancer rates, encourages the frequent use of olive oil.

- **Polyunsaturated fats:** There are two or more double bonds and even fewer hydrogen atoms in this fat type. These are also liquid at room temperature. Polyunsaturated fats, which our bodies are not capable of making, are divided into omega-6 and omega-3 fatty acids.

  Note: Almost a century ago scientists discovered that by chemically altering polyunsaturated fats using a process called partial hydrogenation, a liquid vegetable oil can be made into a solid, thus becoming easier to ship. This process creates what are called trans-fats. Trans-fats, such as margarine and Crisco, are a nutritional disaster! They should be avoided not only to protect your breasts but also to safeguard your heart and brain.

Omega-6

Omega-6 essential fatty acids are found in polyunsaturated vegetable oils such as corn, safflower, soy, and sunflower oil. These essential fatty acids are required for regulating your metabolism, decreasing inflammation, maintaining your reproductive system, and enhancing your body's immune response. Their chemical structure is dictated by the location of the double bonds within the fat molecules.

Omega-6 fatty acids are everywhere in the American diet. While omega-6 fatty acids are not inherently harmful, it is the imbalance between the omega-6 and omega-3 fatty acids that is unhealthy. Properly balanced, they confer many health benefits.

I prefer to describe the omega-6/omega-3 association as a Dr. Jekyll and Mr. Hyde relationship. Let me explain.

In the cells of the body, non-reactive (or inert) omega-6 fatty acid is converted into more reactive downstream fatty acid metabolites. Much like the conversion of certain hormones such as estrogen, it is the metabolites, not the parent, which have the most biologic activity. The omega-6 fatty acid chemical pathway includes the conversion of linolenic acid to gamma-linolenic acid and subsequently dihomo-gamma-linolenic acid. Food sources of gamma-linolenic acid include evening primrose oil and slow-cooked oatmeal.

When dihomo-gamma-linolenic acid is formed, your body must decide whether to use it to make the anti-inflammatory prostaglandin 1 (PG1) series hormones or the arachidonic acid-induced inflammatory hormones. Your body requires both to defend itself and remain in optimal working condition. This is why omega-6 fats are essential for life. The appropriate intake of omega-6 in conjunction with omega-3 fatty acids (the omega-6 to omega-3 ratio) directs dihomo-gamma-linolenic acid to form a healthy balance of these two types of hormones, PG1 and arachidonic derivatives. This is the Dr. Jekyll side of omega-6.

Studies have found that the optimal omega-6 to omega-3 ratio is 4 to 1. Unfortunately, the standard American diet wreaks havoc on this ratio. Instead of the 4 to 1 ideal, our diets have ratios that range from 10 to 1 to 20 to 1 or even higher. These excessive levels of omega-6 fatty acids can lead to the production of overwhelming amounts of arachidonic acid-based inflammatory hormones, which can increase the risk of cancer, heart disease, and other ailments of aging. This is omega-6's Mr. Hyde side.

Factors leading to the overproduction of arachidonic acid include high dietary levels of omega-6, insufficient dietary amounts of omega-3, and elevated insulin levels. Studies investigating the effects of excess fat ratios have shown that they increase the risk of breast cancer by 87 percent.

Omega-3

Omega-3 fatty acids are the good fats. Found primarily in seafood, flaxseed, green leafy vegetables, fish, canola oil, and walnuts, omega-3 fatty acids reduce the incidence of cancer, depression, heart disease, rheumatoid arthritis, and a host of other all-too-common degenerative diseases. Unlike omega-6, omega-3 in the standard American diet is deficient.

Omega-3 fats are able to block both the growth and spread of breast cancer cells. The EPA (eicosapentaenoic acid) constituent in omega-3 serves as a "braking system" for arachidonic acid-derived hormones by inhibiting their excess conversion from omega-6 — a very important factor in decreasing inflammation and protecting the breast. The DHA (docosahexaenoic acid) component along with the omega-3s found in flaxseed increase the production of the breast cancer-killing 2-hydroxyestrogen. The downstream metabolites of omega-3 are, for the most part, inactive when compared with those of the omega-6s.

An abundance of omega-3 is found in the oil from deep cold-water fish such as wild salmon, herring, mackerel, and sardines. Based on studies showing that omega-3 reduces the risk of dying from heart disease, the American Heart Association now recommends eating fish on a regular basis. (Inuits and other populations who consume high levels of fish have a very low incidence of breast cancer.)

Other common maladies such as depression and have been linked to an inadequate intake of omega-3, while the aches and swollen joints associated with rheumatoid arthritis have been reduced using omega-3.

The FEM Centre Nutritional Plan is designed to maintain your hormonal balance by providing the proper balance of dietary fat — 20 to 30 percent of your calories should be derived from dietary fats including monosaturated fats such as olive oil, along with foods rich in omega-3. This should create an ideal omega-6 to omega-3 ratio of 4 to 1.

The following list is a recommendation of the types of breast-healthy oils you should incorporate into your daily diet.

Oils for Cooking

- Unrefined (extra virgin) olive oil (medium–low heat)

- Unrefined sesame oil (wok, sauté)

- Unrefined coconut oil (all temperatures)

- Macadamia oil (high heat)

- Grape seed oil (medium-low heat)

- Ghee, which is organic, clarified butter (low heat)

- Organic peanut oil (wok, stir-fry cooking)

Oils for Salad Dressings and Marinades — Store in dark, opaque containers in refrigerator away from light and heat. Use within thirty days.

- Unrefined almond oil

- Unrefined pumpkin seed oil

- Unrefined hemp oil

- Unrefined flaxseed oil

- "Oleic" sunflower oil
- "Oleic" safflower oil
- Unrefined walnut oil
- Unrefined avocado oil

Medicinal Oils — Serving size: 1 to 2 tablespoons for cooking, dressings, and supplementation (no more than twice daily).

- 4 to 1 ratio of unrefined sunflower to flax oil
- Unrefined flaxseed oil
- Organic evening primrose oil (hexane-free)
- Organic borage oil (hexane-free)
- Organic black currant oil (hexane-free)
- Omega-3 fish oil (1.5 to 3 grams daily of EPA+DHA with protein foods)
- Organic unrefined pumpkin seed oil

Note: Adequate intake of B vitamins, zinc, magnesium, and lipase will ensure proper utilization of the above oils within the body.

Nuts and Seeds — Serving size: small Dixie cup (approximately 2 ounces)— one to two servings daily

Nuts and seeds are high in unsaturated fats, minerals, vitamins, and enzymes. They are a great source of protein but they contain many calories and complex carbohydrates, so don't exceed serving size! Use raw, unsalted or lightly toasted. Also, use as flour.

- Almonds
- Walnuts

- Brazil nuts
- Pecans
- Macadamias
- Cashews
- Sesame seeds
- Sunflower seeds
- Pumpkin seeds
- Caraway seeds
- Pistachio

Nut and seed butters are acceptable and recommended. These butters are great in salads and for snacks. Use sparingly: 1 to 2 tablespoons per serving, no more than twice daily.

3. Salt, Food Additives, Caffeine, and Coloring Agents

Salt

To function properly your body needs minerals just as it needs vitamins, enzymes, oils, and water. But again, balance is key. An excess of minerals can be dangerous to your health.

Salt (sodium chloride) is a frequent additive in most processed foods, and on average, Americans consume much more than is necessary. Excessive salt intake can aggravate high blood pressure, creating additional work for the heart and kidneys. Many people are unknowingly sensitive to salt. The good news is, with a bit of patience and willpower, you can slowly wean yourself from excessive salt use and reduce this unnecessary strain on your vital organs.

Decreasing your salt intake will reduce the loss of calcium through your urine. In fact, halving the amount of salt you ingest doubles the amount of calcium that remains in your body and is safer than having to take calcium tablets to prevent bone loss.

Food Additives and Coloring Agents

Each year, Americans consume more than 100 million pounds of coloring agents, artificial sweeteners, and preservatives. These food additives are designed to prevent spoilage or enhance flavor, but many have been linked to diseases such as depression, asthma, sensitivities/allergies, hyperactivity, and migraine headaches.

The federal government has banned the use of several of these synthetic chemical additives, but many more remain on the market and in the foods we eat every day. Many people assume that if the government approves it, it must be safe. This is a dangerous hypothesis, because it often takes years for damaging effects on the body to become apparent to research scientists.

Most consumers would balk if offered a teaspoonful of chemicals with names like sodium benzoate, nitrite, monosodium glutamate (MSG), or aluminum, but they seldom hesitate to devour these chemicals when they are included in a brightly colored, overly processed "convenience food."

Caffeine

Caffeine belongs to the methylxanthine family and is a stimulant commonly found in our diet. The effects of caffeine on the breast have been controversial, but most studies agree that it worsens fibrocystic changes. On numerous occasions, I have seen women's breasts dramatically improve after stopping or drastically lowering their intake of caffeine.

The link to breast cancer is not clear. A large study performed on a group of Swedish women showed no association with breast cancer incidence. Still, I have concerns about the role of caffeine in breast health and hormonal balance:

- Fibrocystic changes of the breast can result in atypical cell growth, which is associated with breast cancer. Caffeine has been shown to increase atypical growth.

- Caffeine can block breast cells with damaged DNA from self-terminating. This is particularly worrisome if other genetic defects are also present, such as BRCA1 or BRCA2 mutations.

- The continuous stimulant effect of caffeine tends to promote adrenal gland exhaustion. This will lead to imbalances in cortisol, DHEA, and adrenaline.

I realize that many of us depend upon that cup of coffee or tea every morning to start out the day, but one should attempt to decrease caffeine intake to the lowest tolerable level.

Action Items

Obviously, the more highly processed the food, the more chemical additives it will contain, so reading labels is the foremost advice I can offer. Additives and agents to avoid include:

- Coloring agents such as FD&C yellow dye #15 (also known as tartrazine), yellow #6, and blue #1 and #2

- Monosodium glutamate (MSG)

- Preservatives such as BHA, BHT, tBHQ, sodium benzoate, nitrates, nitrites, and sulfides. These have been linked to cancer and/or allergic reactions

- Aspartame (sweetener)

- Reduce caffeine intake

4. Water (Nature's Best Medicine) and Beverages

The human body is 70 percent water. Water is the single most important substance your body needs to function properly. Water is an essential component of blood, which transports cells and nutrients throughout the body while removing toxins. At some point, every process and activity your body undertakes is dependent upon water. This we all know.

But did you know that water helps to metabolize stored fat? To rephrase the adage about the apple and the doctor, "Eight glasses of water a day helps keeps the fat away." Here is how it works:

The liver and kidneys are designed to filter toxins from your blood. But the liver is also the organ that converts stored fat into usable energy. An ample supply of water keeps both the liver and kidneys functioning properly. If you "turn the water off," the kidneys become less effective at their job, leading to a concentration of toxins.

The body responds by transferring some of the kidneys' workload to the liver. This additional burden causes the liver to reduce its fat conversion process. The result: More fat remains in the body and weight loss is reduced or stops altogether.

As we have seen before, without the correct "balance," the body cannot function as it was designed. Plumbing, whether in your body or your house, needs to be kept open, flushed, and free of obstacles, and water is the simple, inexpensive key.

What about water retention? Ironically, drinking plenty of water actually tends to minimize water retention. When the body gets too little water, it begins to perceive a threat to survival and tries to store every precious drop. Water is stored outside the cells, showing up as swollen feet, legs and hands. The body holds onto water in order to dilute toxins. (An increase in toxins therefore leads to an increase in water retention.) This compensating mechanism is how the body protects itself. The solution to pollution is dilution.

Man-made diuretics offer a temporary solution to excessive water weight but they do this by forcing the kidneys to remove water. A side effect of this process is the loss of essential nutrients along with the water. For this reason, diuretics can be harmful and should not be used for weight loss. (As an alternative, I recommend natural diuretics such as dandelion root, grapefruit, or cranberry juice.)

Action Item

The many pesticides, pollutants, and chemical treatments such as chlorine and fluorine detract from the positive effects of water and are to be avoided whenever possible. Pure water is ideal, but often hard to obtain. Bottled water usually tastes better than most urban tap water, but ideally, you should investigate installing a water filtration system for your home, they come in a wide variety of styles and prices.

Recommended Beverages (daily intake)

- Water — six to eight glasses daily (reverse-osmosis, mineral-enhanced)

If you're overweight, drink one additional glass of water for every 25 pounds of excess weight. Since a larger body has a greater metabolic load and since water is the key to fat metabolism, an overweight person will benefit from additional water.

To avoid excessive snacking during the day, drink eight ounces of water at the first sign of hunger. If hunger persists after twenty minutes, it's probably time to eat.

Increase your water intake during exercise and/or exposure to hot weather. You can easily become dehydrated without realizing it, especially after forty minutes of aerobic exercise.

- Decaffeinated, organic black tea — 1 cup

- Organic green tea — 3 cups

- Organic herbal teas (counts as water) — 3 cups

- Decaffeinated, water-processed organic coffee — 1 cup

- Non-starchy vegetable juices — 8-ounce serving daily
  - Wheat grass
  - Spirulina
  - Barley grass
  - Chlorella
  - Kamut
- Fresh-squeezed fruit juice — 4- to 6-ounce serving
- Cranberry concentrate with water and stevia
- Lemonade (fresh-squeezed with water and stevia)

Sweeteners

- Stevia (liquid or powder)
- Lo Han
- Agave nectar
- Splenda (the jury is still out on this, so use sparingly)
- Xylitol (preferably from birch instead of corn)

Condiments

- Apple cider vinegar
- Organic mustard
- Balsamic vinegar
- Seaweeds
- Rice vinegar
- Braggs Liquid Aminos
- Organic ketchup

- Nasoya

- Wheat-free low-sodium soy sauce

- Follow Your Heart vegenaise

- Rapunzel organic vegetable bouillon cubes

- Eden Foods miso paste and powdered packets

- Fresh, organic herbs

- Homemade marinades

Beverages to Avoid

- All soft drinks (diet or not)

- Milk, milkshakes

- Anything containing high-fructose corn syrup

- Anything containing aspartame (Equal, Nutrasweet)

- Alcohol

- Beer

Note: Red wine may be used occasionally, limited to one glass.

5. Determine Calories for Your Optimal Weight

A calorie is a unit of measurement used to express the heat-producing or energy-producing values of a particular food. In diet discussions, calories are often used as a unit of energy or indirectly as a quantity of food that can be consumed. Both contexts are correct and appropriate.

Your metabolism receives calories through fats, carbohydrates, and proteins, which differ in their caloric values. The primary sources of calories are carbohydrates and fats. The highest calories occur in fat; the most readily accessible calories are found in carbohydrates, and calories from proteins are used by the body only as a last resort under extreme conditions, i.e., starvation.

Studies show that location and amount of fat cells in your body are important. Visceral adipose tissue is fat that is located primarily around the waist area. It gives you the shape of an apple. This fat is dangerous for the breasts as well as the heart and brain. A healthier location for fat seems to be in the hip area. This type of fat distribution creates more of a pear-shaped body profile.

If you divide your waist measurement by your hip measurement you get your waist-to-hip ratio. A ratio of less than 0.8 is breast-healthy, with the ideal being 0.74. A ratio greater than 0.85 increases your risk for breast cancer and other degenerative diseases.

One of the best ways for reaching and maintaining optimal health and wellness is through calorie restriction. In test after test with different animal species, restricting calories resulted in a longer life with less breast cancer and other chronic disease.

As we grow older, restricting calories is particularly important. It is crucial that you adjust your diet when you reach midlife. Your metabolism slows while your hormones go through many changes. As we age, we often fail to realize that we cannot eat the same types or amounts of food as we did in our twenties or thirties.

Calorie restriction does not mean malnutrition, diet pill-induced fasting, or fad starvation diets. You should eat enough food to maintain your health while avoiding excess calories. There are two components to weight control: weight loss and weight maintenance. Weight loss requires taking in fewer calories than you burn daily. For most women this translates to less than 1,500 calories per day. After reaching a desirable weight, calories can then be adjusted appropriately.

In a standard American diet, the most important foods to minimize relative to calories are carbohydrates. Eating carbohydrates in the proper quantity allows your body to better regulate blood sugar and reduce the production of damaging free radicals.

Successful restriction of calories requires balancing the dietary centers within the brain. Being overweight can be thought of as a disease resulting from imbalances of the master neurotransmitters serotonin and norepinephrine. Neurotransmitters are proteins that are stored in the brain and subsequently released by nerve endings in order to transmit chemical messages to other nerves. As with hormones, a neurotransmitter deficiency means that the message stops and health problems occur.

Without proper instructions, your appetite becomes uncontrolled, leading to additional ingestion of food and resulting in weight gain. Mood changes resulting from neurotransmitter imbalances can initiate stress and contribute to the release of weight-inducing hormones such as cortisol. Adequate levels of serotonin tend to limit sweet and chocolate cravings, while sufficient amounts of norepinephrine decrease the overall desire for food.

Four main causes of neurotransmitter deficiency include:

- Stress

- Toxins

- Poor nutrition

- Prescription drugs for depression, anxiety, or appetite suppression

Our breast care program offers solutions for each of these causes including stress reduction, removal of toxins, and a nutritional plan that restores neurotransmitter levels.

A deficiency in serotonin and norepinephrine results not only in weight issues, but it also underlies the current epidemic of depression and anxiety. To understand the magnitude of this problem, we need look no further than estimates showing that as many as 30 million Americans take antidepressants. Prescription antidepressants such as Paxil, Prozac, Zoloft, Celexa, Wellbutrin, and Lexapro, over a period of time, might actually worsen neurotransmitter deficiencies.

In a similar fashion, the use of appetite-suppression drugs, which include phentermine and Tenuate, can do more harm than good by worsening long-term weight control.

Relying on the eight years of experience that NeuroResearch Clinic's Marty Hinz, M.D., has accumulated in the treatment of almost twenty thousand patients, I recommend that specific amino acid supplementation combined with certain vitamins and minerals be used for the restoration of serotonin and norepinephrine. The amino acid 5-hydroxytryptophan (5-HTP) is converted into serotonin, while chemical reactions convert L-tyrosine to norepinephrine. (These two amino acids are generally deficient in the American diet.) Nutrients that facilitate these reactions (cofactors) include vitamins B6, B12, C, folic acid, and calcium. If you suffer from low levels of serotonin and norepinephrine, studies have revealed that to replenish them, you may require a daily dietary intake of approximately 300 milligrams of 5-HTP and/or 3,000 milligrams of L-tyrosine. To obtain these amino acid levels in the body, one would have to eat eighteen egg whites or forty ounces of red meat daily. Instead, I suggest that these two amino acids and their cofactors be obtained in the form of supplements.

Action Items

Daily caloric intake depends upon your frame size, height, ideal weight, and activity level, but in general, to achieve anti-aging benefits from caloric reduction I recommend:

- Caloric restriction – approximately 1,200 calories daily (if a lower intake, such as 1,000 calories, is required, please be followed by a health care provider) until desired weight is achieved, then caloric maintenance

- Do not consume more than 500 calories at any meal

- Do not skip meals, especially breakfast

- Eat every three to four hours, including a late-afternoon and evening snack of protein bars
- Drink a glass of water before each meal
- Avoid fast foods
- Balance neurotransmitters using 5-HTP and L-tyrosine

Do not become discouraged when trying to implement these suggestions; it takes about three weeks of practice to retain good, new habits. (See the *Twenty-Minute Eating Rule* in Appendix C.)

CHAPTER 8

Detoxification: The C.A.N. Program and Chelation

Fatigue, weight gain, insomnia, memory loss, joint and muscle aches, cold and heat insensitivity, and the general feeling that "things are not like they used to be" occur with increasing frequency as women enter their midlife years. Attempts to address only these symptoms employing hormonal balancing frequently result in frustration and less-than-optimal results. An increased buildup of toxins in the body can also account for these symptoms. Detoxification must first be accomplished to enhance the effectiveness of hormonal balancing. I believe that the goal of a detoxification program should be threefold: 1) to avoid breast cancer, 2) to diminish the incidence of chronic disease; and 3) allow for the proper balancing of your hormones.

Detoxification, whose significance generally has been overlooked in traditional medicine, is an important physiologic function that deals with how toxic waste is disposed of by your body. Basic goals of detoxification include: 1) the removal of toxins from the cell and its surrounding matrix, 2) the chemical conversion of these toxins into less harmful metabolites, and 3) the subsequent excretion of these metabolites from the body.

Toxins can be thought of as substances that interfere with the optimal function of your body. The toxins that are formed inside you are "endogenous." Endogenous toxins originate from daily cellular metabolism, which involves the use of hormones and the chemical interaction of oxygen and glucose to produce the energy needed to run the cell. Resulting exhaust products of energy production, known as free radicals, can easily damage a cell's DNA. In addition, breakdown products, or downstream metabolites, of hormones such as estrogen have been shown to be very toxic, especially to the breast.

We all are toxic to some degree, thanks to our heavily polluted environment. Toxins are acquired by daily exposure to environmental (exogenous) pollution including industrial sludge, heavy metals, pesticides, radiation, hydrocarbons, and food additives.

The total amount of toxins that your body either generates or absorbs is referred to as the *toxic load*. Studies show that failure to detoxify and reduce the toxic load can add to the risk of contracting breast cancer and the other chronic diseases of aging. Aging, along with poor dietary habits and lifestyle choices, can result in an increase in the toxic load that your body has to process. An excessive toxic load can act on several levels:

- Creating an overactive immune system, which results in chronic inflammation leading to destruction of the cell matrix and injury to the cell;

- Suppressing the immune system, which inhibits the body's ability to watch for and protect against cancer;

- Disturbing hormonal balance.

To understand the magnitude of your detoxification needs, realize that your body consists of some 70 trillion cells. Since each cell generates toxic products, you have as many as 70 trillion trash cans to empty every day.

In a large city where sanitary services have been disrupted, the lack of waste removal results in the accumulation of piles of trash (an urban toxic load) accompanied by a rapid deterioration in living conditions. If your body is not able to empty its trash cans and excrete this waste, you can expect to see a like deterioration in your living condition (health).

Those parts of your body that come into contact with the outside world and therefore are especially exposed to toxic insults include the digestive system, the respiratory system (lungs and nose), and the skin.

The intestinal part of the digestive system is particularly vulnerable. Because of its large surface area (approximately that of a tennis court), the intestines can be exposed to enormous amounts of potentially toxic substances. Almost 30 tons of ingested material will pass through the digestive system in an average person's lifetime. While the intestines' goal is to selectively absorb life-sustaining nutrients while rejecting the rest, a breakdown in the protective intestinal barrier allows unwanted foreign material or toxins to leak into the bloodstream. This leakage can increase the risk of breast cancer.

The lymphatic system and blood vessels function as the waste management trucks that ultimately must carry not only these pollutants but their by-products to waste processing centers such as the liver and kidneys. From here they are excreted from the body either by the colon or in the urine.

How do you know if you have a toxic overload? We have provided a basic questionnaire (Appendix A) to give insight into your current state of toxicity.

The Cellular Matrix

As seen in Figure 9, hormones travel through the bloodstream and pass through what is called the *cellular matrix*. As you age, more and more toxins collect in this cellular matrix. Since these toxins are chemically active, this accumulation interferes with the function of hormones as they seek to interact with each cell.

In fact, a cellular matrix, when overloaded with toxins, acts much like a clogged filter in a home's air conditioning system. You can replace your air-conditioning unit, but until you clean the air filter, no amount of tinkering is going to increase its efficiency. That is why physicians can tell you, "But your hormones are fine!" when you feel terrible. Doctors are actually measuring the hormones in your bloodstream, and have no idea what the level of hormones may be in your cells.

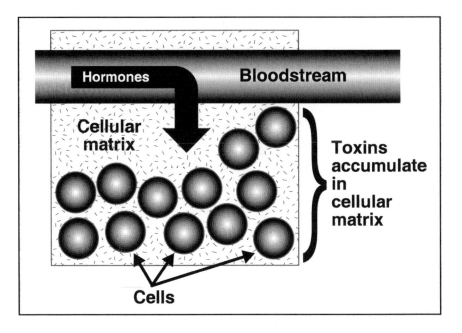

Figure 9. *The endocrine hormonal pathway.*

Hormones provide indispensable biological information to your cells. If their paths are blocked or compromised, this information will not be properly delivered. Without it, your cells will not know when to stop dividing, nor will they interact properly with their neighbors, thus giving rise to a malignant environment.

The goals of our Breast Care Program are to reduce inflammation and keep estrogen at safe levels within the breast by means of detoxification. Detoxification reduces the body's toxic load and promotes breast health by:

- Lowering the risk of injury to cell DNA.

- Regenerating the cell support structure, the cell matrix.

- Maintaining the integrity of the body's cancer surveillance system.

Food and the Second Brain

Food, the most important medication in our daily lives, provides essential information to the body. This information is supplied in the form of water, vitamins, minerals, nutrients, enzymes, and other items needed to allow your body to allocate resources and maintain long-term health. This food "information" enters your body through your digestive system.

Some doctors refer to the digestive system as the "Second Brain" because it processes the incoming information provided by food like the "First Brain" processes incoming data provided by the senses. To take this analogy a step further — the Second Brain can receive a constant stream of harmful information in the form of poor food choices and environmental toxins like the First Brain can be polluted by constant exposure to such toxic information as dismal news reports, violent movies and video games, and pornography.

The digestive system begins with the mouth, teeth, gums, and salivary glands. Most of us fail to realize how vital this area is to our overall health. A mouth that contains amalgams, root canals, and gum disease provides fertile ground for the development of chronic inflammation and heavy metal contamination. Pregnant women with poor dental health have been shown to have a higher risk for premature labor.

Root canals and gum disease provide points of chronic infection that promote generalized inflammation throughout the body. Studies have implicated chronic periodontal inflammation in heart disease, stroke, and diabetes. Dental amalgams used in tooth cavities can be a primary source of pollution from such heavy metals as tin, mercury, and nickel. I, along with other researchers, have documented sometimes significant electrical activity between amalgams and the adjacent gum tissue. This activity essentially allows heavy metals to cross over into your bloodstream.

Good dental health is a great starting point for cutting your toxic load and eliminating sources of chronic inflammation. Daily brushing and flossing cannot be overemphasized and are essential for reducing the possibility of dental disease and promoting overall good health.

The next part of the digestive system consists of the stomach and the intestines (which is further subdivided into the small intestine and colon).

The stomach's highly acidic environment limits bacterial growth within it. However, as we age, the stomach environment can become less acidic permitting the excessive growth of *H. pylori (Helicobacter pylori). H. pylori* is a major cause of stomach ulcers. This overgrowth of bacteria, in turn, further lowers the acidity of the stomach, resulting in indigestion, heartburn, and an inadequate breakdown of food before it passes into the small intestine, affecting various hormones, particularly insulin. Rapid dumping of partially digested food into the intestines causes an excessive secretion of insulin, subsequent hypoglycemia, and worsening of inflammation throughout the body.

The intestines are the heart of the digestive system and the primary immune organs of the body. Both digestion and protection from the outside environment rely on maintaining a friendly relationship with bacteria that colonize the entire digestive system. One's ultimate health and avoidance of cancer (especially breast cancer) can depend upon this symbiosis.

The small intestines contain more bacteria than the stomach but the majority, by far, is found in the colon. The colon contains a complete ecosystem containing some 100 billion bacteria divided into more than 400 different species. Bifidobacterium and lactobacillus, which we make use of in our gut restoration program, are regarded as two of the most beneficial bacteria lining the colon. These bacteria not only interact with the food you eat to create beneficial nutrients that feed the intestinal cells but also help balance the immune system. Little wonder that a breakdown in this finely tuned relationship is a major contributor to the chronic diseases of aging.

The intestines also serve as a barrier to the infiltration of environmental toxins. With time, this barrier can become porous or leaky, allowing an influx of toxic elements into the bloodstream. This is commonly known as "leaky gut syndrome." A constant intestinal leakage of toxins activates the immune system, which can elicit symptoms of chronic inflammation such as fatigue, joint pain, muscle aches, fuzzy memory, eczema, psoriasis, and asthma. Chronic inflammation leads to tissue destruction, and if allowed to go unchecked, can produce permanent harm to tissues such as the brain, heart, bones, and breasts.

The health of the colon can play a key role in determining the risk of breast cancer. Traditional medicine is just beginning to accept this connection. Studies have shown that prolonged use of antibiotics may double the risk of breast cancer. The relationship between antibiotics and the health of the intestines is a possible explanation for this finding.

The chronic use of antibiotics alters the healthy flora of the intestines, allowing disease-causing elements to set up house. Without the proper symbiotic relationship between the good bacteria and the cells that line the intestines (colonocytes), leaky gut syndrome allows toxins to enter the bloodstream, activating the body's immune system and leading to chronic inflammation. This inflammation can affect breast cells in the following manner:

- The cell matrix can be disrupted by inflammation, allowing the breast cells to become disconnected from their neighboring cells and to divide uncontrollably.

- Inflammation leads to an increase in DNA mutations in the breast cell, especially to those genes that stop uncontrolled division.

- Inflammation activates enzymes such as aromatase that produce excessive amounts of estrogen that lead to overstimulation of breast cells.

Note: Instead of using antibiotics as an example, we could have substituted food allergies, parasites, hydrocarbons, pesticides, heavy metals, or any number of other potential insults to the intestinal lining, that promote hormonal disruption. And instead of citing damage to the breast, we could have cited the brain, heart, bone, joints, skin, etc. This reinforces the underlying point of our Breast Care Program — what protects the breasts will also protect the heart, brain, and bones.

Liver-Intestinal Detoxification System

After crossing the intestines, substances are carried to the liver by the portal blood vessels. This forms the liver-intestinal detoxification system, which is responsible for filtering and removing the majority of toxins that enter the body from the outside.

The liver performs many duties, including: 1) removing and neutralizing toxins; 2) modulating the immune system; 3) metabolizing hormones such as estrogen; 4) controlling clotting factors; and 5) metabolizing fats, carbohydrates, and even proteins. Each of these is influenced by intestinal function.

As the intestines become porous from continued exposure to the standard American diet, the liver is faced with more toxins to neutralize and the need to place the immune system on high alert. External toxins such as plastics, antibiotics, pesticides, and petroleum products are broken down by specific enzymes (CYP450) inside liver cells. If one has a genetic predisposition to poor enzyme function, or the level of toxins is so great as to overwhelm the capability of these enzymes, the liver cannot adequately neutralize these harmful agents and may even suffer damage itself. Toxins will then be dumped back into the bloodstream, traveling to all parts of the body (a condition known as toxemia).

The connection between an environmental toxin, liver detoxification status, and breast cancer risk was shown by a group of researchers who in 1996 published an article in the *Journal of the American Medical Association* entitled "Cigarette smoking, N-acetyltransferase2 genetic polymorphisms, and breast cancer risks." Genetic analysis revealed that a certain group of women are born with a lower level of activity of a specific liver enzyme that is required to break down a toxic byproduct (carcinogenic aromatic amines) of cigarette smoke. The medical term for these women would be "slow acetylators." Tracking a group of postmenopausal women who were both slow acetylators and smoked more than one pack a day revealed a 4.4 times increased risk of breast cancer. There was no increase in breast cancer for those who smoked the same amount and length of time but had normal liver enzyme function.

Other factors that diminish the effectiveness of the liver detoxification enzymes, such as pharmaceutical medicines (cimetidine, acetaminophen) and alcohol, add to one's breast cancer risk. A woman who has a combination of deficient liver detoxification enzymes and genetic risk factors such as the mutated BRCA genes or poor methylator genes could be at even greater risk for breast cancer.

Combined high level toxic exposure (especially heavy metals) in conjunction with eating too many processed foods containing inadequate amounts of healthy nutrients will finally impact the ability of the liver to support its detoxification enzymes. Important nutrients that support liver function include N-acetylcysteine (NAC), lipoid acid, selenium, and the herb silymarin. These are discussed in Appendix B.

The liver also modulates the body's responses to infection and inflammation. Remember that an estimated 75 percent of the body's immune system resides in the intestines, which are referred to as the gut-associated lymphatic tissue, or GALT. A breakdown of the intestinal lining, or leaky gut, can activate the intestinal immune system, which releases inflammatory chemical messengers (cytokines) that travel to the liver. Inside the liver are specialized cells known as Kupffer cells which are really white blood cells. Almost 10 percent of the liver is composed of Kupffer cells. The intestinal-derived inflammatory messengers, upon reaching the liver, will instruct the Kupffer cells to generate more inflammatory chemicals, which will be transported by the bloodstream to all areas of the body, including the breast.

This can be thought of as a relay team at a track meet in which a runner from the intestines, with a baton containing instructions for generating inflammation, races to the next relay station, which is the Kupffer cell. As the baton is passed off to the Kupffer cell, hundreds, even thousands, of new runners are generated, carrying these batons throughout the body to other relay stations located in the breast, heart, and even brain. Relying on the initial signal from the intestines, the liver then amplifies the message of inflammation. Should this occur on a continuous basis, we then have chronic inflammation, which is a major cause of the diseases of aging.

The liver responds to increased inflammation by producing more of the anti-oxidant, cholesterol.

If the friendly bacteria that line the intestines are replaced by less friendly bacteria, candida, or parasites, a similar process of continuous amplified inflammation occurs. Candida not only produces estrogen-like compounds that are hormonal disruptors, but also releases part of its fungal wall, which is quite inflammatory. Similarly, hostile intestinal bacteria can excrete inflammatory lipopolysaccharides to incite the liver. Chronic inflammatory changes eventually can disrupt the surrounding environment of the breast cell and lead to excessive estrogen production. Long-term use of antibiotics — through the adverse alteration of the normal intestinal bacterial flora — can double the risk of breast cancer.

Metabolism of estrogen that circulates in the bloodstream takes place primarily in the liver. Enzymes (CYP450) used in this process differ from those found in the breast cell. The goal of the liver is to prevent the excess buildup of the body's total estrogen load. Estradiol is converted to estrone, which then is metabolized into 16alpha-hydroxyestrone or 2-hydroxyestrone. Very little 4-hydroxyestrone is made in the liver unlike the breast. 16alpha-hydroxyestrone is then converted into estriol, which along with the methylated version of 2-hydroxyestrone is chemically packaged in order to be excreted into the urine or bile. These estrogen metabolites then enter either the colon or will pass through the kidneys and out the bladder. Nature has designed a remarkably efficient system of disposal. Interruptions to this system by the absorption of toxins such as xenoes-trogens, and by bowel irregularities, commonly lead to estrogen im-balance and overstimulation of the breast cell.

A leaky gut allows for the increased absorption of xenoestro-gens, which include the organochlorine chemicals (PCBs), non-organochlorine chemicals (hydrocarbons), heavy metals (cadmium), and agricultural hormones found in animal products. These envi-ronmental hormonal disruptors have the ability to hamper the de-toxification of estrogen by overwhelming or inhibiting liver enzyme function.

Problems that arise when estrogen is delivered to the colon include irregular bowel habits, particularly constipation, and the overgrowth of bacteria containing the enzyme beta-glucuronidase. Constipation al-lows estrogen to remain for a longer time in the intestines, increasing reabsorption. Beta-glucuronidase releases estrogen from its binder molecules, permitting reabsorption back into the body. Overgrowth of the bacteria containing beta-glucuronidase can lead to elevated levels of the enzyme and a rise in blood levels of estrogen.

Hormonal balancing is also influenced by the intestinal-liver in-teraction with orally administered estrogen replacement. This as-sumed particular importance in the WHI study and explained many of the adverse reactions including increases in blood clots and strokes. When estrogen (either synthetic or bio-identical) is swal-lowed by mouth, it will be absorbed through the intestinal lining into the bloodstream and transported to the liver. This "first-pass" phenomenon results in different effects as opposed to the same hor-mone passing through the skin and initially missing the liver.

The first-pass interaction of estradiol with the liver results in 1) a large portion of the estradiol being converted to estrone; 2) a sulfate molecule being added to the estrogen, inactivating the hormone but increasing its water solubility; 3) an increase in sex hormone-binding globulin and other hormone binding proteins; 4) activation of factors that increase blood clots, which can lead to strokes; 5) a lowering of cholesterol but not triglycerides; 5) an increase in the inflammatory marker high-sensitivity C-reactive protein (hsCRP); and 5) a change in bile consistency, which may increase the risk of gall bladder disease.

The liver also plays a major role in the metabolism of carbohydrates, fats, and protein. Storage, conversion, and absorption of these basic nutrients are biochemical functions that are interwoven with the intestines. It is the regulation of insulin by the processing of carbohydrates and fats in the intestines that is important for breast health.

The liver-intestinal detoxification system is key to hormonal balance and breast health. Each of the two organs depends upon the other for proper functioning. A breakdown in this system leads to persistent chronic inflammation, which paves the way for chronic disease including breast cancer.

Symptoms that are linked to liver-intestinal detoxification problems include bloating, indigestion with heartburn and belching, irritable bowel syndrome (alternating constipation and diarrhea), and gallbladder disease.

Figure 10 illustrates the chain of events that can occur in the intestines and lead to health problems.

A woman should begin detoxification (as well as hormonal balance, described in Chapter 9) as early in life as possible, but it's especially important to implement these actions during the first few years after the onset of menopausal symptoms. What happens then has a long-term effect on her health.

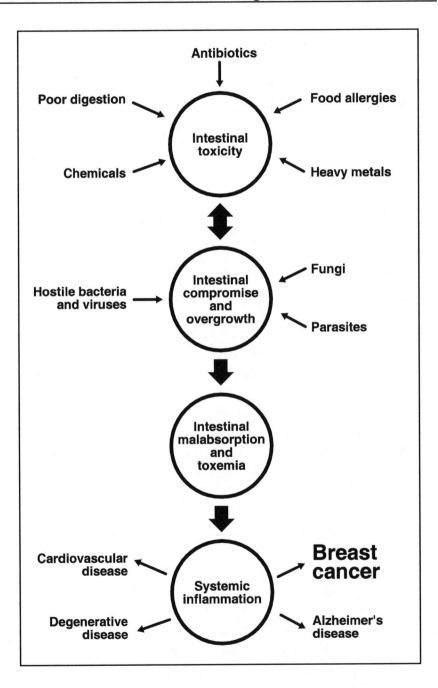

Figure 10. *The chain of events related to intestinal problems.*

The C.A.N. Program (*Cleanse*, A*dd*, N*ourish*)

The first step in correcting a leaky gut and re-establishing proper function of the liver intestinal detoxification system is to cleanse the gastrointestinal tract by eliminating unhealthy substances that have accumulated there. These may include:

- Harmful bacteria

- Viruses

- Fungi

- Parasites

- Allergens

- Toxins

A health-care provider well-versed in detoxification is your best asset in eliminating these hindrances to intestinal health. Treatment can sometimes require specialized testing and medications, along with supplemental nutrients.

Dietary changes also can be effective in removing toxins and allergens, and practicing what is known as an *oligoantigenic diet* can be very useful. (An oligoantigenic diet is one containing only those foods known to pose a low risk for allergic reaction.) Formal food allergy testing may be necessary to help determine the proper oligoantigenic diet. Again, the physician can assist you, although you'll also find a breast-healthy detoxification diet in Appendix B.

Disease-causing agents such as yeast, molds, viruses, parasites, and bacteria also have to be considered. They can colonize anywhere in the intestinal tract and can affect the immune system, creating symptoms not easily traced to a specific cause or agent.

Finally, examining and discussing your history with the doctor often can identify exposure to external toxins or noxious agents such as perfumes and pesticides that may interfere with good intestinal health.

The next step is to *add* desirable biological components that establish a proper balance of microbes in the newly cleansed gastrointestinal tract. These may include:

- Hydrochloric acid

- Digestive/pancreatic enzymes

- Beneficial bacteria

Hydrochloric acid and pancreatic enzymes, which tend to decline as we age, are important to the digestive process. They ensure adequate breakdown and absorption of fats, proteins, and carbohydrates.

The addition of beneficial bacteria is accomplished by the reintroduction of desirable bacteria known as probiotics. These bacteria produce various vitamins and short-chain fatty acids required for the colon's cell growth and function. They also break down toxins and prevent colonization by disease-causing agents — this is probably their most important function. The small intestine requires the proper bacterial flora such as acidophilus while the large intestine also requires bifidobacterium.

The final step is to *nourish*. Once you have cleansed your gastrointestinal tract and added beneficial bacteria and other digestive aids, you must continue to maintain this fragile balance. This is accomplished with direct nutritional support using:

- Fiber (prebiotic)

- Vitamins

- Minerals

- Antioxidants

- Amino acids — such as glutamine

- Butyrate

In most instances, some healing of the intestinal tract by maintaining the colon's floral colonies is required to restore proper function. Glutamine and butyrate help with this healing, since they are the preferred fuels for the rapidly replicating cells of the gastrointestinal lining. They are especially helpful with problems caused by stress, injury, sepsis, and inflammation. A lack of glutamine is associated with atrophy and degenerative changes in the small intestine, while butyrate similarly supports the large intestines.

Other co-nutrients such as zinc and vitamin C are also important to the nourishing process. Zinc is crucial to the control of irritable bowel syndrome, and vitamin C helps control the *H. pylori* bacteria.

Establishment of good bowel habits, along with proper hydration, cannot be overemphasized, since estrogens and their metabolites 2-hydroxy, 4-hydroxy, and 16alpha-hydroxyestrogen are ultimately excreted either into the intestines or urine.

Weight control can also be realized through detoxification. Many women experience a ten- to fifteen-pound decrease in weight simply following the C.A.N. program and saying "no" to wheat and sweets.

As we have stated before, fat cells produce estrogen and inflammatory chemicals, which can act to initiate and propagate breast cancer cells. Being overweight (twenty to seventy pounds above your optimal weight) can double to triple your risk of getting breast cancer. Being overweight is a greater risk for breast cancer than taking Prempro!

Case Study: Detoxifying After Breast Cancer

Susan is a breast cancer survivor. At age 44 she had a right breast lumpectomy and was diagnosed with invasive ductal cell cancer of the breast. A modified mastectomy and courses of chemotherapy and radiation followed. Her oncologist placed her on the drug tamoxifen.

The four years since breast surgery had not been easy. She had struggled with premature menopausal symptoms resulting from her cancer treatment. The fatigue, hot flashes, joint and muscle pain, anxiety, insomnia, and weight gain were overwhelming. A recent MRI had indicated significant fibrocystic changes and other worrisome signs in her left breast. The oncologist even mentioned a possibility of ductal carcinoma *in situ* (DCIS). Now 50, Susan was looking for a change in direction and came to the FEM Centre.

Susan's problems — years of water retention, bothersome food sensitivities, bloating after eating, 30 percent body fat, signs of intestinal candida overgrowth, elevated homocysteine blood levels, and a score of 13 on the FEM Centre Detox Questionnaire — were consistent with poor digestion and underlying chronic inflammation. Two issues needed to be resolved: 1) address and remove the symptoms she is currently experiencing, and 2) prevent the recurrence of her breast cancer. Aggressive detoxification and restoring her liver-intestinal detoxification system was the answer to both.

She decided to stop tamoxifen and commenced taking breast care nutrients including iodine and a supplement containing DIMN (diindolylmethane), calcium D-glucarate, and red wine extract. She started our Cleanse, Add, Nourish program that included the 21-day detox diet. Digestive enzymes -- amylase, proteinase, lipase and betaine -- were added to her meals along with a probiotic composed of various strains of bifidobacterium and lactobacillus combined with minerals and medicinal oils.

During the first two months her bloating was alleviated and her swelling resolved. Gradually, her joint and muscle pain disappeared. Further cleansing removed any residual intestinal candida or parasites. By the sixth month her body fat was just 21 percent and her detox score was 3. Her homocysteine levels were declining, and her body was better able to methylate.

A repeat MRI showed a noticeable decrease in fibrocystic changes and a marked improvement in the overall pattern of blood flow in the breast. Hot flashes were significantly reduced, and her ability to sleep had improved. The result: "I can't believe that I really feel this good," she said. "My energy has finally returned."

Chelation Therapy

A frequently ignored but important component of detoxification that is required for breast health is accounting for and removing the heavy metals that have accumulated in your body. These metals include arsenic, cadmium, lead, mercury, tin, nickel, and aluminum. Of particular concern is cadmium, which has been found in high concentrations in breast tissue. It can act as a hormonal disrupter by mimicking the action of estrogen.

How do you acquire these heavy metals? The answer is that we live in an industrialized society where heavy metals have been released into the environment for decades. Cadmium is found in cigarette smoke and seepage from batteries. Aluminum is acquired from cookware, deodorants, and the water supply. Dental fillings, eating fish such as tuna, or playing with a broken thermometer as a child all are avenues for mercury to enter the body. Arsenic is found in the water supply, tobacco products, and certain types of pressure-treated wood. The lead from fuel and paint products that were removed from the market years ago still resides in the bones of those who lived during that era. (Scientists have found levels of lead in the bones of modern-day people 500 to 1,000 times those found in people who lived in the 17th century.)

Heavy metals, upon entering the body, eventually find their way into the cellular enzyme system, where they can disrupt function by forming very strong ionic bonds. Enzymes are essential for the proper operation of the cell. Inhibiting the functioning of these enzymes will eventually result in catastrophic events within the cell, making it useless or even cancerous. If heavy metals disrupt the enzymes of cells that compose the immune system, early stages of cancer can go unchecked by this primary defense system.

Heavy metal exposure is everywhere and has been found to be a factor in the majority of the chronic diseases of aging. Studies have revealed that small amounts of lead released from menopausal bones can result in high blood pressure. In order to remove heavy metals that have become trapped within the cell and its matrix, one must use *chelation therapy*.

Chelation, which is derived from the Greek word for "crab," is a well-studied medical practice for removing toxic metals. It makes use of special molecules (chelators) that have a strong electrical affinity for metal ions. The chelator surrounds the heavy metal molecule to form a chemically inert (or biologically inactive) molecular complex that is then excreted into the urine or colon.

Nature has provided us with natural chelators including vitamin C, cysteine, and glutathione. However, we must rely on more powerful chelators, such as ethylenediaminetetraacetic acid (EDTA), dimercaptosuccinic acid (DMSA), and dimercaptopropanesulfonic acid (DMPS), to extract those metals that are deeply bound in our cells.

While much attention has been paid to the positive effects of chelation in relation to heart disease, the therapy's ability to boost the body's immune system against cancer also shows promise. A study was performed by Drs. Brummer and Cranton involving a community in Switzerland that underwent chelation treatment and was medically followed for almost twenty years. A significant reduction (90 percent) in both cancer- and heart-related mortality was noted among those who were chelated as opposed to those who were not. As part of a long-term breast care program, we recommend chelation to all women, especially 40 years and older.

Before one embarks upon a chelation program, a urine provocation test is required to identify which heavy metals are present. Blood level tests are not always helpful since heavy metals lodge deep within the cell and its matrix. The urine provocation test is performed by administering either one or a combination of chelation agents, followed by collection of urine for a period of six hours. The specimen is then sent to a special laboratory where it is analyzed for the types and amounts of heavy metals present. (We believe this to be a superior method to simply performing a hair analysis.) The type of chelation agent that is needed can then be determined.

Midlife women need to incorporate chelation therapy into their wellness plan not only for cancer prevention, but also for protection against chronic diseases of aging, such as eye diseases (macular degeneration), heart disease, neurological disease, dementia, and Alzheimer's. (In the bibliography, books have been listed which further explain the benefits of heavy metal removal.)

A simple way to reduce the body's heavy metal load is through the use of an oral chelation program. Intravenous routes are generally reserved for specific medical conditions such as heart disease. A physician who has been trained in chelation therapy should supervise your treatment program.

We have found that using an oral preparation of liposomal-encapsulated EDTA for twenty-five to thirty weeks can result in dramatic drops in heavy metal concentrations. Once this has been accomplished, periodic dosing every three months prevents metal re-accumulation.

Additional Therapies

Detoxification can be enhanced by far-infrared sauna treatments, colonic therapy, homeopathic drainage remedies, and traditional Chinese medicine. These therapies assist in ridding the body of stored toxins.

A **far-infrared sauna treatment** uses heat to penetrate tissues. This aids in the excretion of toxins from within your fat cells by "sweating" them out.

Colonic therapy involves more than receiving an enema. A trained colon therapist uses a specially designed apparatus to irrigate the colon. While flushing the toxins that reside in both the intestines and the liver-gall bladder system, colonics can reduce parasite, fungal, and bacterial overgrowth. Colonics can also replace essential nutrients.

Homeopathy, which is based on the concept that "like treats like," provides various remedies that enhance the body's ability to remove toxins. This is often accomplished through an enhancement of lymphatic drainage.

Traditional Chinese medicine relies on the use of both herbs and the energy conduits of the body known as meridians. We have had great success in detoxification using a combination of these techniques.

Additional Tests

In most cases simply using the FEM Centre cleansing program achieves adequate detoxification. Should the need arise, other methods are available to detect and quantify the body's toxic load. Most of these tests measure the effects that toxins have on the body and not the actual toxin levels. These tests include:

- C-reactive protein test
- Complete digestive stool analysis (CDSA)
- Organic acid/dysbiosis analysis
- Food sensitivity testing
- Biocellular analysis (BCA)
- Bioimpedance analysis (BIA)

Chronic inflammation is a common manifestation of toxic buildup. A blood test, which initially was used to measure acute inflammation but now has been shown to reflect chronic inflammation, is the **high-sensitivity C-reactive protein** (hsCRP) test. The liver is stimulated by inflammatory substances, namely interleukin-6, to synthesize hsCRP. Multiple chronic diseases of aging including heart disease and Alzheimer's have been linked to elevated levels of hsCRP. Although this test does not point to the exact cause of the inflammation, many health-care providers recommend this screening procedure.

The **complete digestive stool analysis** evaluates the health of the intestinal tract by measuring several markers for digestive and absorptive ability. It also reflects the intestinal levels of the enzyme beta-glucuronidase, which can impact breast health.

The **organic acid/dysbiosis analysis,** obtained by examination of a urine specimen, measures metabolites generated by energy production, brain functions, and unwanted intestinal organisms.

Food sensitivity testing using blood samples can help isolate problematic allergy symptoms (itching, rash, even shortness of breath) and delayed toxic reactions (headaches, fatigue, irritable bowel, eczema) due to the food you ingest. Gluten, a component of wheat, has been increasingly linked to many of these symptoms. Food sensitivity testing provides one of the few ways to identify those women who should avoid gluten. More severe cases of gluten sensitivity can result in celiac disease.

The FEM Centre program also makes use of two tests that provide an objective measure for monitoring the progress of those who follow our detoxification program: biocellular analysis (BCA) and bioimpedance analysis (BIA). Biocellular analysis provides data on the body's acid/base balance by measuring the pH levels of the blood, saliva, and urine. Establishing an optimal alkaline environment provides for the healthy function of a cell's chemistry, while an acidic environment promotes chronic diseases and hormonal imbalances. Because of the ability of the BCA to measure mineral and electron concentrations, it is possible to evaluate oxidative stress levels, adrenal function, and mineral status.

Bioimpedance analysis is a total body measurement that extends from hand to foot. It is performed by passing a small electric signal between electrodes attached to different parts of the body in order to measure changes in voltage and current strength. This allows for an accurate determination of the amounts of lean muscle mass, fat, and the percentage of intra- and extracellular body water. As toxicities increase: 1) water shifts from inside to outside the cell, while 2) a decline in lean muscle mass with a subsequent increase in fat tissue (most often seen with aging and lack of exercise) further aggravates the body's hormonal balance. Multiple studies involving cancer and AIDS patients have confirmed the accuracy of the BIA in determining body composition and response to medical treatment. Both the BCA and BIA help to determine the degree of toxicity as well as provide objective procedures to monitor the effectiveness of the FEM Centre program.

With advances in genetic research in the last ten years, a great deal of attention is now being focused on an individual's genetic makeup. The ability of the body to break down toxins into non-toxic substances relies, for the most part, on its genetic blueprint. A certain portion of the human population has genes that are inefficient in producing these detoxifying enzymes. This leads to toxin accumulation and the potential for an increased risk of chronic disease. Genetic screening using either blood or salvia samples can pinpoint potential weaknesses in your ability to detoxify. These tests are readily available at a health practitioner's office specializing in detoxification. While the FEM Centre program is designed to overcome these deficiencies, knowing that you have this genetic predisposition should be a prime motivator to help guide your lifestyle choices.

The components of the FEM Centre's approach to detoxification, the C.A.N. program and chelation therapy, are meant to optimize your digestive system, cleanse your toxin filters, and raise your overall health I.Q. in the process.

CHAPTER 9

Balancing Hormones

Approximately 1 million American women enter menopause every year, and these women are inundated with often-contradictory information that deals with hormone imbalance, hormone replacement, supplementation, and depletion.

Most people think our hormones decline or become imbalanced as we become older. Contemporary anti-aging medicine has reversed that concept — we become older because our hormones decline or become imbalanced.

Balanced hormones are important to maintaining breast health, so it's vital to sort through the mountains of research data, uninformed opinions, and marketing campaigns to achieve a proper understanding of the latest research and its implications for achieving hormonal harmony.

The underlying concept is that *no hormone should be used by itself.* Instead, a balanced combination is required to achieve overall health while avoiding breast cancer. This is one problem with the WHI study, which looked only at a single hormone replacement. Each hormone is interdependent, acting in concert with the others to counter the effects of aging and to foster optimum health.

It is also important to recognize that it is not just the hormone that produces biologic changes, but also the hormone's downstream metabolites. In fact, these metabolites may have more profound biological effects than the hormone itself.

With the approach of menopause, one may notice physical and psychological changes. Your health and sense of physical and mental well-being are directly linked to these hormonal imbalances. The restoration of this balance can help reverse or at least slow the detrimental effects of aging.

Some scientists estimate that twenty to thirty years of "youthfulness" can be added with proper hormone replacement. Ten to fifteen years is a more conservative estimate, but in either case, the positive health effects of balanced hormones cannot be overestimated.

Responses to hormonal deficiencies vary with each individual. Some women might experience only one or two symptoms, whereas others may suffer from a wide range of negative effects. Symptoms resulting from estrogen deficiency include:

- Hot flashes and night sweats

- A decrease in energy

- Fuzzy memory

- Unexplained weight gain

- Changes in skin texture

- Mood swings

- A decrease in sex drive

- Sleep disturbances

Medical science has created a longer average life span (not necessarily a longer health span) for today's woman. Our aging society is seeing an epidemic of cancer, dementia, Alzheimer's, and other debilitating effects. But, on the positive side, research in the fields of endocrinology and immunology has increased our knowledge of how and why we age, and offered new and better ways to enhance our quality of life.

Hormone production begins to decrease in midlife and diminishes in an almost linear fashion, causing a decline in the body's ability to self-regulate its functions and adapt to its environment. These changes can contribute to the subsequent onset of chronic diseases such as heart disease, neurological diseases, cancer, diabetes, arthritis, and various autoimmune problems. Restoring hormones to an optimal balance helps re-establish this self-regulation and adaptation.

The Effects of Hormones

Before deciding on proper balancing, we need to understand the concept of hormones and how they work. Hormones regulate your body's energy production, temperature, growth, immune system, reproductive capabilities, and neuroactivity.

Hormonal balance is influenced by your lifestyle, eating habits, the state of your liver-intestine detoxification system, and the function of your endocrine glands (the ovaries, adrenals, and thyroid). Genetics, the environment, and life experiences (which are influenced by social and cultural factors) also play a role. This means that a special hormone plan is required based on the needs of each individual. There is no one-size-fits-all approach to hormonal balance.

A hormone is a molecular messenger that acts on adjacent cells (paracrine), or within the cell that generates it (autocrine), or travels throughout the body to sensitive tissue sites (endocrine).

While some scientists adhere to the classical description of a hormone binding to a receptor as a key fits into a lock, others believe that a hormone can resonate with a specific cell receptor without coming into direct contact — much like a radio station's signal resonates only with a specific type of antenna. The antenna then carries the signal to a radio just as a resonating cell receptor evokes a response from its target cell. As a result of this "resonation" effect, each cell can be in communication with trillions of other cells in your body. This would explain how hormones, which are found in such minute quantities in the bloodstream, could affect so many important functions.

A blockage in the flow of hormonal information results in stagnation of biologic information. Prolonged stagnation leads to a decrease in your body's self-adaptation and regulation, which then gives rise to chronic disease. However, in certain cases, instead of a blockage in the flow of information, there may be a flood of information, again giving rise to disease. *The key is balance!*

As a rule, you should avoid the use of synthetic hormones for replacement. Instead, use only bio-identical hormones.

When considering hormones and the use of supplements, we must also distinguish between the terms *deficiency* and *insufficiency*. Traditional medicine tends to recognize deficiency, which is really the end stage, or ill effects, that are the result of an insufficiency. It is best to try to correct insufficiencies rather than wait for deficiencies to develop.

There are several ways to assess hormonal levels: saliva, blood, and urine. The specific hormone determines the method of measurement. For most hormonal evaluations, blood sampling is sufficient. Regardless of the method that is used it must be remembered that the resultant hormonal levels are, at best, an indirect measurement of what is really present inside the cell itself, especially that of the breast.

Saliva is a blood filtrate, which is supposed to contain the unbound or free hormone. There are questions as to the validity of saliva testing regarding:

- How to store for shipping

- How to correlate levels after replacement hormones are administered

- How to correct for diet

Our experience has shown that saliva tests can be used to screen for certain hormonal imbalances but are not particularly helpful in monitoring or adjusting hormone replacement doses. In the majority of cases, we prefer blood sampling for hormonal assessment. Saliva testing should be considered only in those for whom hormone blood levels cannot be obtained, who require the measuring of melatonin and cortisol, and for those perimenopausal women who need serial hormonal measurements obtained throughout their menstrual cycle (generally eleven samples). Urine collection is more cumbersome in our experience, but can be useful especially in the evaluation of cortisol.

The body has designed a system of checks and balances to prevent too much hormone from entering a cell. When interpreting hormonal levels, especially that of blood, one must consider the role of sex hormone binding globulin (SHBG). Sex hormone binding globulin is a protein that is made in the liver and binds to most of the estradiol in your blood, essentially inactivating it. Not only does SHBG act as a transport for estradiol in the blood, but it also keeps it from entering the cell. This is of particular importance in preventing breast cancer, by limiting the amount of estradiol that can enter a breast cell. Women with higher levels of estradiol and lower levels of SBHG have been shown to be at greater risk for breast cancer. Conversely, if SHBG levels become too high, free estradiol levels are lowered to the point that one experiences symptoms of estrogen deficiency.

There are many factors that influence levels of SHBG — insulin, low-fat foods, dietary fiber, vegetable products, exercise, and oral ingestion of estrogens (especially synthetics).

Human growth hormone (HGH) and thyroid hormones also have specific binding proteins, HGH binding globulin and thyroid binding globulin (TBG), which if increased to excessive levels, tend to lower the effective amounts of these important hormones. Bio-identical and especially synthetic oral estrogens can result in an elevation of these binding proteins.

Labs determine hormonal ranges using averages based on a large sampling of women to identify deficient or excessive levels. The resultant normal range is usually wide. For instance, the total T3 (the active thyroid hormone) has a normal range from 85 to 205 picograms per milliliter (pg/mL). Technically, if you were at 85 pg/mL, traditional medicine would consider this to be in the normal range. The real question is, "Do you feel normal?" Or are you suffering from symptoms that go untreated because your lab considers your data to be in the low range of the "normal" category?

There is a definite decline in the quality of life for those in the lower 25 percent as opposed to those in the upper 25 percent of the "normal" hormone range. I have yet to encounter a laboratory that asks how you feel at 85 as opposed to 170 pg/mL. At 85 pg/mL, you would not be deficient but might suffer from insufficiency, depending upon symptoms such as fatigue, dry skin, cold hands and feet, weight gain, and hair loss.

The optimal approach is to try to raise your hormonal levels to that of a 25-year-old woman, which in this case would be a total T3 between 170 to 205 pg/mL — the middle to upper normal range for most lab standards. Most women in midlife will notice a vast improvement in symptoms using this approach to hormone balancing.

Balancing multiple hormones using this rationale will result in an exponential increase in well-being and health as opposed to, say, concentrating on estrogen alone without consideration of the other hormones mentioned in this chapter.

While a number of different hormones are made by your body, optimal health and wellness can be achieved by balancing the following hormones:

- Estrogen (also see Chapter 3 — Estrogen Explained)
- Progesterone
- Testosterone
- Pregnenolone
- DHEA
- Thyroid
- Melatonin
- Cortisol
- Insulin
- Human growth hormone (HGH)

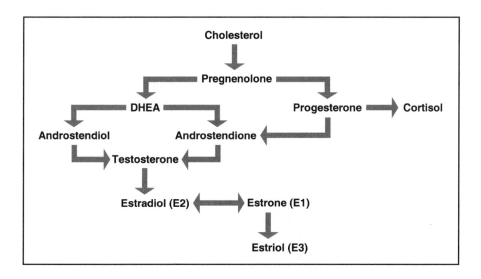

Figure 11. Cholesterol-derived hormone pathways.

Many of these hormones have a common precursor — cholesterol. Figure 11 illustrates the pathways from which various hormones are derived from cholesterol.

Estrogen Applications

Note: My outcome-based clinical observations, along with recent findings of the WHI, confirm the health benefits of estrogen replacement. However, the type of estrogen, the amount, and the route of administration, along with adherence to the FEM Centre Breast Care Program, are significant considerations when using estrogen replacement therapy.

The FEM Centre Breast Care Program uses various combinations of the three natural estrogens: estrone, estradiol, and estriol. Using natural, or bio-identical, hormones is crucial in hormone replacement therapy. These hormones are safer than synthetic hormones and are derived from vegetable sources. Each of these hormones is used individually or combined in ratios depending upon an individual's needs. Common formulations include:

- Individual doses, usually of estradiol or estriol, but rarely estrone;

- Combinations of two, called *biest* — with *bi* indicating two estrogens;

- Combinations of all three, called *triest* — with *tri* indicating three estrogens.

Biest

Biest most often consists of estradiol and estriol. A common, weak formulation of biest is 20 percent estradiol to 80 percent estriol. This mixture is good for women who require only a small amount to address symptoms. For those with greater needs, a stronger recommended ratio could be ⅔ estradiol to ⅓ estriol.

Because natural estrogens tend to break down over a twelve- to fourteen-hour period, single dosages of biest should be taken first thing in the morning, and for the lower doses, one also at bedtime. Biest preparations can be applied directly to the skin, sublingually (under the tongue), or orally.

Triest

Our breast care program views triest as the most advantageous estrogen combination. Estriol, when combined with estradiol and estrone, tends to have the benefit of protecting the breasts from potential cancer formation.

Common ratios of triest, which I make use of, range from the lower strength of 80 percent estriol, 10 percent estrone, 10 percent estradiol (80/10/10) to the stronger dosage of 30/20/50. There are an infinite number of combinations to use. The blood levels of estradiol that need to be achieved with triest are well within the "normal" range for a menopausal woman. Our experience suggests that most women will have an estradiol level of 20 pg/mL to 50 pg/mL after taking triest.

Triest is best applied transdermally as a cream or gel. (When taken orally, a significant amount of estradiol is converted to estrone in the liver, reducing its effectiveness.) A transdermal application enters the bloodstream directly, allowing estrone to act as a reservoir for conversion to estradiol as the body requires. Other advantages of transdermal applications are:

- Fibroids do not seem to grow.

- Blood vessels undergo more relaxation, allowing for a normalization of blood pressure.

- Incremental adjustments can be made according to one's needs. (With pills, patches, or pellets, one size must fit all.)

- Estrogens bypass the liver, avoiding higher risks of blood clots, strokes and heart disease.

- The lowering of circulating levels of triglycerides.

- No lowering of thyroid hormones or human growth hormone (again, because the liver is bypassed).

- Less effect stimulating breast tissue, studies have indicated, and possibly better protection against colon cancer.

Note: Transdermal triest used in combination with our breast health program does not increase the incidence of breast cancer.

Optional methods of application are patches applied to the skin surface; pellets placed under the skin; troches and drops, which dissolve either in the mouth or under the tongue (sublingual); and pills or capsules, ingested orally.

Patches containing bio-identical estradiol are available by prescription under such trade names as Vivelle and Climara. Patches have some disadvantages versus creams and gels. A patch does not contain the buffering effects of estriol and estrone, and only comes in predetermined doses.

Troches are similar in composition to gels, but are dissolved either under the tongue or between the cheek and gum. Levels of estrogen tend to peak rapidly and are not evenly distributed throughout the day.

Pills and capsules have some disadvantages. Because they initially pass directly through the liver, estrogens are transformed into metabolites before reaching the cells in your body, which can decrease the amount of estrogens available. Other hormones can be reduced by these actions, including thyroid and human growth hormone.

Key Observations on Estrogen Replacement Therapy

Our clinical study of almost 2,300 women (some of them perimenopausal, most of them postmenopausal) who followed our breast care program over a five-year period provides verifiable data that estrogen replacement therapy can be both beneficial and safe. No breast cancers were reported in those who used transdermal triest preparations. Only one breast cancer without metastatic spread occurred in a postmenopausal woman, who is currently disease-free. The breast cancer rate in our study is much lower than would be expected even in women who did not take estrogen. Incorporation of the FEM Centre Breast Care Pyramid was key to this success.

The results of the WHI study agree with our clinical observations and act as a guide for *what not to do.*

Breast tissue makes over twenty times more estrogen than that found in blood levels of postmenopausal women not on estrogen replacement. Combined with the estrogen made by your fat cells, this represents the greatest danger to your breasts.

Measuring estrogen in blood, saliva, or urine does not necessarily reflect the internal environment of the breast cell. Currently there are no available methods outside a research setting to exactly measure estrogen and its metabolites in the cell. Reports that suggest postmenopausal breast health can be determined using complex formulations of urine or blood levels, such the estrone + estradiol / estriol, must therefore be viewed with caution.

Proper estrogen replacement is determined by the type, amount, and route of administration. One must account for the breakdown and proper disposal of estrogens that you either make or take.

Many women express confusion over the issue of weight gain and estrogen. Estrogen has what is described as a bimodal effect on weight gain. Too little estrogen in the body causes the cells to become less sensitive to insulin, which leads to weight gain. Without estrogen, muscle-building, calorie-burning hormones such as testosterone are ineffective. As a result of low estrogen, women who enter menopause often suffer from an increase in fat about their midsection.

Conversely, elevated estrogen levels also result in weight gain because of excessive cell stimulation. This causes water retention and increases fat in the breast and hip areas. In between these two extremes, optimal levels of estrogen can actually help one lose weight. This is readily accomplished using the hormone-balancing program described in this chapter.

Gel/Cream Application

When using gels or creams, avoid the breast. Apply to areas of the body that allow the best absorption, where blood vessels are closest to the skin surface, such as the inner arm (especially upper part), wrist, ankle, and inner thighs. A larger surface area allows for greater absorption. Rub in fifteen to twenty times to ensure proper application, and do not wash the area for at least thirty minutes.

Estrogen Symptom Summary

Excess: Breast tenderness and enlargement, water retention and bloating, irritability, worsening of PMS, weight gain, heavy or abnormal uterine bleeding, fibrocystic changes in the breasts, growth of fibroids, initiation and promotion of hormone-dependent cancers.

Deficiency: Hot flashes, night sweats, vaginal dryness, frequent urination, decrease in sex drive, fuzzy memory, depression, weight gain, changes in skin and breasts, osteoporosis, accelerated aging, increase in heart disease, increased risk of cancers such as colon cancer.

Progesterone

Progesterone should be considered part of a hormonal balancing program in any postmenopausal woman, regardless of the presence of a uterus. Progesterone is the hormone produced in the ovaries of menstruating women. It is also made by the placenta during pregnancy. Thus it derives its name from the Latin *pro* meaning "for," and *gest* meaning "gestation." (Although progesterone is made primarily by the ovaries, a small amount is derived from the adrenal glands, which are small glands near the kidneys.)

In addition to sustaining pregnancy, progesterone assumes the role of a hormonal harmonizer. It acts as a "braking system" for estrogen. Unlike estrogen, your body can never overproduce progesterone naturally. In fact, during pregnancy, levels reach more than twenty times those found post-ovulation, and even then, those levels are not considered excessive.

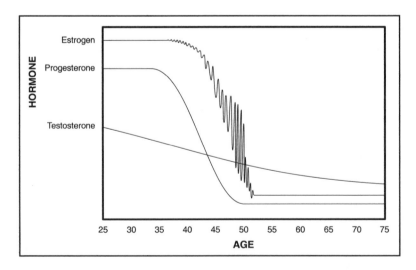

Figure 12. Estrogen/progesterone/testosterone levels during life transitions.

A woman's initial hormonal transition is estrogen dominance (Figure 12), which most often results from a decrease in progesterone. Progesterone, not estrogen, is the first hormone that begins to decline dramatically prior to menopause.

Heavy bleeding, fibroids, tender breasts, water retention, and even endometriosis are common manifestations of estrogen dominance. Inadequate progesterone is a major contributor to each of these conditions. In our experience with routine vaginal sonography, we estimate that up to 50 percent of women in this hormonal transition have fibroids. Combine fibroids with excess estrogen and lower progesterone, and one has heavy menstrual flows.

Many important physiological actions are attributed to progesterone, including:

- Helping prevent cancer of the breast and uterus

- Supporting the uterine lining and sustaining pregnancy

- Normalizing blood clotting mechanisms

- Stabilizing moods

- Reducing anxiety

- Decreasing night sweats

- Acting as a natural diuretic

- Increasing good cholesterol (HDL)

Contrary to what many have been led to believe, progesterone is heart-healthy. Administration of progesterone to women with heart disease undergoing an exercise stress test reduces the incidence of angina, or heart-induced pain.

Clinical studies have revealed that progesterone may assist in new bone formation, but the exact mechanism is not clear. This would explain why premenopausal women who do not ovulate, but still produce estrogen, can still suffer bone loss.

After passing through the liver, progesterone may be metabolized into allopregnenolone, which has a sedative effect. This is believed to be an anti-anxiety hormone that levels a woman's moods. Taken in the evening, progesterone can provide relaxing and sleep-enhancing effects. Postpartum mood changes ranging from "the blues" to deep depression can also respond to progesterone therapy.

Stress and anxiety lower progesterone by causing the continual release of cortisol from the adrenal glands. If this persists, the adrenals must tap their resources, which involve the diversion/conversion of progesterone into cortisol.

To compound the problem, these mood upheavals can lead to mixed signals sent from the brain to the ovaries (as shown in Figure 5, Chapter 5), inhibiting ovulation and further decreasing progesterone. Thus begins a vicious cycle — lower progesterone allows estrogen to dominate, leading to irritability, anxiety, and mental stress, which can lead to even lower levels of progesterone.

Progesterone Misconceptions

There is a common misconception in most hormone replacement programs — women who do not possess a uterus are told they no longer need progesterone. In fact, it is the opposite — if you begin estrogen replacement therapy, you should also use progesterone, whether you have a uterus or not.

Another major misconception has resulted from various studies and the news media's alarmist reports of such studies. Most studies involve the use of synthetic progesterone (such as Provera). Progestins are the family of hormones which technically include natural (bio-identical) progesterone but most often refer to the synthetic versions. A progestin can produce negative results such as reversing the positive effects estrogen has on the heart and the cardiovascular system. And while progesterone inhibits breast cell division, certain progestins do not.

Synthetic progestins also cause new blood vessels to grow inside the uterus, particularly in the uterine lining. This can cause spotting or breakthrough bleeding in women on hormone therapy.

This is an important distinction to make when considering results of studies that focus only on synthetic progesterone. Natural progesterone doesn't cause such problems, and is rarely used exclusively in these studies. In fact, progesterone decreases the ability of estrogen to bind to cells such as those in the breast, which prevents overstimulation, often a precursor to breast cancer. In contrast to the negative effects of progestins on the cardiovascular system, natural progesterone relaxes smooth muscle cells, whether in the uterus or the lining of blood vessels.

Progesterone, like estrogen, is metabolized by the breast cell into downstream metabolites, which play important roles in controlling cell division. The two main metabolite groups include the 5α-pregnanes and the 4-pregnanes. Studies by Dr. Wiebe have revealed that the 4-pregnanes are the primary cancer-inhibiting hormones, which decrease cell division and increase cell adhesion preventing metastasis. 5α-pregnanes seem to have the opposite effect.

Progesterone Application

As with estrogen, bio-identical progesterone is recommended. Progesterone can be administered via cream, capsules, liquid, or troches placed under the tongue. (Injectable forms exist, but have a limited role outside of infertility treatments.) The exact dose varies according to route of administration.

Progesterone must be taken daily in moderate quantities to have a protective effect on the breast. Initially (the first four to six weeks), the breast may be tender, but this will eventually pass. A series of thermograms taken over a period of time clearly shows that continuous application of progesterone to the breast can result in a resolution of worrisome changes such as fibrocystic disease.

Your choice of application and frequency will depend on what hormonal transition you're experiencing. Premenopausal women may wish to use a cream or oral application for approximately two weeks per month. Menopausal women on estrogen replacement therapy and who still have a uterus will use progesterone daily. In most cases, an oral progesterone preparation is recommended to achieve higher blood levels. Oral progesterone may be started at 50 to 100 milligrams once or twice daily and adjusted to ensure that there is no growth in the uterine lining. Again, it is important to monitor blood levels or vaginal ultrasounds to ensure that the uterine lining is not encouraged to grow, especially if a progesterone cream is used.

Creams should be applied to areas that have a blood supply readily accessible (the inner arm region, back of your hands or wrist) to permit adequate absorption, while avoiding areas with fat such as the abdomen. Usually, for those with PMS or estrogen dominance, a 2 to 3 percent natural progesterone cream of one-quarter teaspoon twice daily beginning at midcycle and extending for no more than two weeks (starting on Day 12 to 14 and stopping on Day 26 to 28) will correct low progesterone levels. If you are experiencing anxiety, oral progesterone seems to work better.

A menopausal woman with a uterus, who is on estrogen replacement, needs a higher progesterone cream dosage than a woman with PMS. Since blood levels do not always correlate with the dosage of cream used, vaginal sonograms are a good idea to monitor the uterine lining.

Some practitioners advocate the postmenopausal use of progesterone in a cyclic fashion, varying between fourteen to twenty-one days with fourteen to seven days off. This is too complicated, hard to remember and, in addition, is questionable for the following reasons:

1. By stopping the progesterone, cells that are found both in the uterus and breast can begin to divide again. Cell divisions in these two organs are not something we want to encourage, especially during postmenopause. Researchers have found that progesterone prevents breast cell division *only* when taken in continual doses. With or without a uterus,

menopausal women gain added protection against breast cancer through daily use of progesterone. "On and off" use of progesterone also allows for the resumption of menstrual flows for those with a uterus and taking estrogen, which would negate one of the benefits of postmenopause — no more flows.

2. Some argue that continual use of progesterone results in abnormal insulin response, causing both weight gain and higher risk of heart disease. While synthetic progestins and the high levels of progesterone seen in pregnancy may result in altered levels of insulin, we have found that bio-identical progesterone, in appropriate doses, does not affect insulin levels over the long term. Research has shown that after six months, insulin levels normalize (even after taking oral contraception).

For the menopausal patient on estrogen replacement, there are several ways to take progesterone:

On a cyclic basis — anywhere from fourteen days to twenty-one days of the month, which can lead to the resumption of menstrual flows.

Daily (preferred) — results in no bleeding by attenuating the uterine lining, and affords the breast maximum protection.

Progesterone Symptom Summary

Excess: Drowsiness, dizziness, depression, low sex drive, delayed or erratic menstrual cycles, increased appetite, weight gain, possible decrease in testosterone levels, exacerbated *candida* growth.

Deficiency: Estrogen excess or dominance, menstrual irregularities, hormonal cancers such as that of the uterus and breast, anxiety, and mood fluctuations.

Testosterone

Testosterone is a hormone known as an androgen, and among androgens, it is the most powerful. Androgens are considered "male hormones," but that designation masks their importance as a necessary part of a female's hormonal balance. Androgens (also known as "anabolic" hormones) are responsible for building and maintaining tissue such as bone and muscle (as opposed to catabolic hormones such as cortisol, which causes tissue breakdown and faster aging).

Testosterone controls the amount of muscle in the body, and that's important since we tend to lose muscle as we age. To add to the problem, when you lose muscle, it's replaced by fat!

Testosterone is also important in increasing one's sex drive, energy, assertiveness, bone density, cognitive ability, and overall well-being. Testosterone also boosts the level of human growth hormone. Many doctors and researchers believe the decline in androgens, which begins in your mid-thirties, ultimately initiates the process of physical aging.

Adrenal glands and ovaries are the primary sources of androgens in women. The ovaries produce approximately one-half of the circulating testosterone, while the other half is derived from the conversion of adrenal androgens by peripheral tissue such as fat cells. Removal of the ovaries will result in a 50 to 70 percent decrease in circulating levels. This explains why surgical removal of ovaries can result in acute androgen deficiency.

Prior to the 1990s, very little attention was paid to the need for androgens in women. Testosterone conjured up visions of hair growth and large muscles. We now know that there is a decline in androgens such as testosterone and DHEA that begins prior to menopause and continues well into postmenopause. Circulating levels are approximately one-half those found during your twenties.

Another reason for a decrease in androgens is oral synthetic hormone replacement. Women who take birth control pills have declines in free testosterone, so avoiding oral estrogen preparations is generally recommended to prevent a decrease in the active hormone levels. (Actually, this includes any oral estrogen preparation, but is especially a problem with synthetic estrogens.)

Testosterone has received a great deal of media attention as the hormone responsible for increasing a woman's sex drive. However, if your sex drive is not what it should be (according to you), testosterone alone will not always be enough. It can often be combined with other hormones, detoxification, and changes in lifestyle and relationships to achieve an overall balance and boost libido. Your lack of sleep, stress, and hormonal changes that your partner may be experiencing should also be considered as factors that can explain a low sex drive.

Testosterone also exhibits protective effects for the breasts. Testosterone is a *prohormone*, which means its primary mode of action is found in the hormones that it is metabolized into, one of which is dihydrotestosterone (DHT). DHT is the most powerful of the natural androgens and acts to protect breast cells by slowing their division. It also maintains cell differentiation, which inhibits potential breast cancer formation.

Some scientists have recommended that including testosterone in any type of hormone replacement therapy for postmenopausal women will reduce any excessive cell division in the breast.

Testosterone Application

Testosterone is available most often as a gel applied transdermally, or as a troche which dissolves in the mouth. (Oral testosterone is rarely used, since it tends to be inactivated by the liver.) As with other hormones, bio-identical testosterone is a necessity, and synthetic preparations are to be avoided.

For long-term application, the cream or gel should be applied in the morning to the inner arm, behind the knee, or above the heel in the area of the Achilles tendon, where there is little hair growth. Always make sure to alternate application sites.

If you notice sexual satisfaction is hampered because of a decrease in clitoral sensitivity, testosterone cream or (non-alcoholic) gel can be applied directly to the clitoris itself and to the labial folds on an alternating basis nightly. This can continue for three or four weeks until sensation has been re-established. Three functions are served: It sensitizes the clitoris, strengthens the muscles around the vaginal opening (including those that support the bladder), and is absorbed into the bloodstream via the venous plexus of the labia. (A mild increase in clitoral size may occur, which acts to increase sensitivity. However, if you notice a marked increase in size, then cease application near the clitoris.)

Other Testosterone Issues

A natural hormone that has been balanced is less likely to have adverse effects; an imbalance can lead to problems. An increase in facial hair growth is one of the most feared side effects attributed to testosterone replacement, but is usually not a problem in replacement programs where blood levels are carefully monitored and normal physiologic ranges are maintained.

Certainly, higher levels (ones we call "supraphysiologic") can result in increased facial hair. Facial hair resulting from testosterone excess is the dark, beard-like hair that is predominantly located on the chin and upper lip. (This is not to be mistaken for the soft white downy hair that is seen on the outer facial areas.) Women who have naturally dark hair with some facial growth may have slight increases that are genetically determined.

Testosterone can increase hair growth in the pubic triangle, since testosterone deficiency may have caused an earlier decrease in pubic hair. On rare occasions, testosterone can cause hair loss on the scalp similar to male pattern baldness; this would also preclude the use of testosterone.

An increase in the secretions of one's sebaceous glands, especially on the face, can result in acne. Women who have such tendencies may notice that testosterone replacement aggravates their acne.

In that case, one should avoid testosterone until the acne is adequately controlled, and then judicious use may be tried. Testosterone use generally should be avoided in women with deep cystic acne because of the potential for scarring.

There are concerns about the effects of testosterone on cholesterol and blood lipids. Studies indicate that high doses of synthetic oral preparations (methyltestosterone) may reduce HDL, the good cholesterol. A safer alternative is bio-identical testosterone given non-orally, which increases blood flow within the heart without adversely affecting cholesterol.

Testosterone Symptom Summary

Excess: Excessive pubic and facial hair growth, minor hair loss, acne, enlarged, oversensitive clitoris, and aggressive behavior.

Deficiency: Fatigue, low energy, loss of sex drive, loss of self-esteem or sense of well-being, a decrease in the ability to orgasm, a decrease in muscle coupled with an increase in fat.

Pregnenolone

Pregnenolone is derived from the metabolism of cholesterol inside the mitochondria of the cell. It has been referred to as a master hormone of aging that is produced in the adrenal gland, ovaries, skin, and nervous system. Pregnenolone is considered a neurohormone.

Most of the research on this hormone has been derived from animals. Some of it concluded that pregnenolone was almost one hundred times more effective in enhancing memory than any other hormone. As a brain hormone, it improves the transmission of nerve impulses while facilitating communication between the brain cells (neurons). Pregnenolone stimulates the excitatory pathways of the brain but if converted into progesterone it indirectly has a calming effect through activation of the gamma-aminobutyric acid (GABA) receptors. We have seen moderate improvement with its use in women who have fuzzy memory. Some experts have recommended that pregnenolone be used to slow the onset or progress of dementia, especially in women aged sixty and older.

The adrenal glands also depend on pregnenolone to function as a building block for the other cholesterol-derived hormones such as cortisol, DHEA, progesterone, and androstenedione (Figure 11, page 137). We have found that levels of pregnenolone are almost always low when DHEA is low.

One of the many important roles of pregnenolone is that it serves as a reservoir for progesterone, DHEA, and cortisol. Chronic inflammation and stress act to drain off pregnenolone in order to increase the production of the stress hormone cortisol by the adrenal gland. This lowering of pregnenolone levels results in an unwanted decline in the downstream production of progesterone and DHEA.

We have found that pregnenolone replacement is helpful in those who suffer from adrenal exhaustion (a depletion of adrenal hormones), and when administered in higher doses, it can help the pain of arthritis.

Studies have indicated that women with breast cancer who did not respond well to endocrine therapy (medicines that block estrogen formation) had a lower rate of conversion of pregnenolone to DHEA than to cortisol. Excess cortisol, a potential promoter of cancer, is being synthesized from pregnenolone, robbing the body of important breast cancer-inhibiting hormones.

Even though there is a decline of about 60 percent between the age of twenty-five and seventy-five, pregnenolone's role in hormone balancing has been a point of debate. While some women have reported improvement in symptoms while taking pregnenolone, others noticed no effect. Until more studies are performed that define specific benefits, we feel that pregnenolone replacement will not be appreciated.

Pregnenolone Application

Common routes of administration include oral; applied to the skin as a cream; or sublingual (dissolved under the tongue). Blood levels should guide the amounts. Oral preparations range from 50 to 150 milligrams daily (although doses of 400 mg daily may be needed for arthritis). A sublingual dose begins at 10 mg daily.

Pregnenolone Symptom Summary

Excess: Since pregnenolone can be metabolized into the hormones listed in Figure 11 (page 137), excessive levels (mainly as a result of overdosing) may result in agitation, acne, oily hair, and fluid retention. However, I have found that aging decreases the ability of pregnenolone to convert to these hormones, minimizing the chance for any of the above side effects.

Deficiencies: Most often trouble with memory but also those symptoms seen with adrenal insufficiency, such as fatigue.

DHEA (dehydroepiandrosterone)

Note: Most of the circulating DHEA in the body has a sulfate attached to it and is referred to as DHEAS, but for simplicity I will use the popular term DHEA.

DHEA was once touted as the miraculous hormone for anti-aging. Many people rushed out to buy DHEA over the counter and took it without medical supervision. But self-administering a single hormone can produce disappointing results. Again, balance is the key to optimizing health.

DHEA is the most abundant hormone in your body and is primarily derived from pregnenolone in the adrenal glands. Levels of DHEA tend to peak in your twenties and by your seventies, DHEA might be as low as 10 percent of your youthful level.

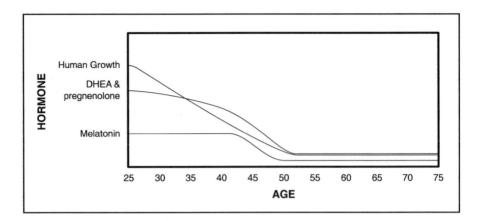

Figure 13. *Human growth hormone, DHEA, pregnenolone,
and melatonin levels during life transitions.*

Obviously, DHEA declines with age and plays a significant role
in the process of biological aging. Stress also takes a toll on the adrenal glands, reducing their ability to produce DHEA. Levels may be
so low that they are not measurable in a woman's initial hormone
assessment.

Low DHEA levels can cause fatigue, fuzzy memory, a diminished immune system, sleep problems, and a constant battle with
weight. Low DHEA can be an indication of adrenal exhaustion,
which is extremely common in women who are affected by the
standard pressures and stress in contemporary society. Without
restoration of the adrenal glands, hormones—especially thyroid—
are very difficult to balance.

On the positive side, DHEA has been associated with:

- Relief of hot flashes

- Elevation of moods

- Controlling obesity

- Building of muscle and bone

- Prevention of cancer

- Prevention of heart disease

- Prevention of non-insulin-dependent diabetes

- Slowing the progression of dementia

- Strengthening the immune system

- Helping in the treatment of systemic lupus erythematosus (SLE)

DHEA counteracts the effects of cortisol on the aging body, especially the brain. DHEA also protects the bones and even the breasts since it is converted into testosterone in the breast cell.

DHEA is considered a prohormone, which means that the downstream metabolites it produces are the primary hormones used by the body. So as you age, DHEA becomes an important reservoir for the production of hormones such as testosterone and estrogen. Should a cell begin to run low on hormones such as estrogen or testosterone, it will obtain DHEA from the bloodstream. Once inside the cell the DHEA can be converted into the appropriate hormone. If blood levels are too low, the cell will have trouble obtaining the required amount of DHEA, leading to hormonal insufficiency. The importance of DHEA is clear: Some 70 percent of premenopausal estrogen and almost 100 percent of postmenopausal endogenous estrogen is derived from the conversion of DHEA. Supplementation of DHEA therefore becomes an important part of hormonal balancing.

Many studies of DHEA have been performed on animals. Claims regarding its use in heart disease have not been verified in human tests. We know that there is no association between elevated DHEA levels and breast cancer risk. DHEA increases natural "killer cell" activity and reduces inflammation. Also, the damaging increase in cortisol levels that occurs with aging can be offset with DHEA.

Androgens such as DHEA may inhibit breast cancer. Clinical evidence reveals a tumor regression in 20 to 50 percent of pre- and postmenopausal breast cancer patients treated with various androgens. A part of DHEA's protective effects occur because DHEA is transformed into androgens such as testosterone within the breast cell. Animals with induced breast cancer that had DHEA levels adjusted to be comparable to a human's exhibited a dramatic inhibition of tumor growth. Some argue that DHEA can also lead to elevated estrogen levels, but current research does not support this. In fact, DHEA has been used in postmenopausal women without stimulating the growth of the uterine lining. DHEA also protects the bones from osteoporosis.

DHEA Application

DHEA can be applied transdermally, most often as a cream, but generally is given under the tongue or swallowed in capsule form. Dosing of DHEA ranges from 5 milligrams under the tongue to between 5 and 100 mg orally. It is advisable to begin on the lower end (around 5 mg in a compounded form) and increase as needed. This generally will prevent acne or other unwanted androgenic side effects. Oral doses greater than 25 milligrams are not usually required.

DHEA is especially recommended for women who have insufficient testosterone levels but do not wish to take testosterone. Your body can then partially metabolize DHEA into testosterone.

DHEA Symptom Summary

Excess (imbalance): Agitation, oily skin (see testosterone).
Deficiency: Lack of energy, immune issues, weight gain (see testosterone).

Thyroid Hormones

Thyroid hormones regulate the body's metabolism, temperature, and cerebral functioning. Located in the lower neck region in front of your windpipe and weighing less than an ounce, the thyroid gland produces less than a teaspoon of hormone yearly. The thyroid makes use of the amino acid tyrosine and iodide to synthesize the thyroid hormones: thyroxine (T4) and triiodothyronine (T3—the biologically active form of thyroid hormone). (Almost 80 percent is T4, while some 20 percent is T3.) Thyroid hormones aid the cell's ability to burn oxygen to produce energy, which is why cold hands, cold feet, loss of hair, dry skin, and fatigue are common symptoms that may be related to a thyroid imbalance.

The thyroid gland acts as an important physical sensor. A biological "canary in a coal mine," it monitors environmental effects on hormone-producing glands, so the status of the thyroid can reflect environmental damage. And, as with other systems in the body, thyroid function declines with age.

The thyroid is subject to two different imbalances: deficiency (hypothyroidism) and overproduction (hyperthyroidism). Currently we are witnessing an epidemic of thyroid disease, especially hypothyroidism, which explains why Synthroid (pharmaceutical thyroxine) is one of the most popularly prescribed drugs. A deficiency in thyroid production is life-threatening.

The brain plays an important role in determining the output of T4 and T3. As hormone levels drop, the brain releases thyroid stimulating hormone (TSH) signaling the thyroid to increase its output of T4 and T3 (see Figure 5, Chapter 5). Since only 20 percent of the body's T3 is actually made by the thyroid gland, the other 80 percent is produced in various tissues such as the brain, liver, kidneys, skeletal muscle, and even brown adipose tissue (fat) by converting T4 to T3.

The body uses three enzymes (D1, D2, D3) to accomplish this. Each is located in a specific cell type and acts to prevent hypo- or hyperthyroidism. The interplay of these three enzymes determines the status of thyroid hormones in your body.

When assessing the thyroid, one should be tested for TSH, total T4, and total T3. Depending upon your symptoms and lab values, thyroid antibodies may also need to be investigated. (Thyroid antibodies interfere with the normal function of the thyroid gland and can lead to hypo- or hyperthyroidism.) Only then can you know what type of thyroid replacement is needed. Measuring only TSH and T4 will not provide a clear picture of the decline in thyroid hormone function.

Many who enter midlife will experience *functional hypothyroidism*. Symptoms are similar to those mentioned for overt hypothyroidism: fatigue, cold hands, cold feet, dry skin, and/or hair loss. Traditional medicine fails to address this condition because lab values generally reveal only a low-normal level of total T3. Functional hypothyroidism occurs most often from the inefficient conversion of T4 into T3 within the cells. The brain is not aware of the lower total T3 levels and therefore does not respond by increasing TSH production. Aging, lack of proper nutrients, and an increased accumulation of toxins are the main causes. In the FEM Centre's clinical experience, detoxification to revitalize the D1, D2, and D3 thyroid enzymes and the addition of natural thyroid hormone replacement have worked well in correcting functional hypothyroidism. Careful monitoring of thyroid hormones can help achieve levels consistent with those of a woman in her mid-twenties.

Determining Basal Metabolism

Proper functioning of the thyroid gland is essential for cells to produce the required energy to maintain optimal metabolic activity. A by-product of cellular energy production is heat, allowing one to maintain a stable body temperature even on cold days. The term "warm-blooded" has even been applied to this biologic evolutionary advancement. The normal range for body temperature is 97.8 to 98.2 degrees Fahrenheit. Many of the body's enzymes and chemical reactions work best in this temperature range. A hypo-functioning thyroid gland or an increase in the body's toxic load can lead to a decrease in cell metabolism that is mirrored by a lower resting body temperature.

A simple way to assess the body's metabolism at rest (basal metabolic rate) can be obtained by measuring the Basal Body Temperature (BBT).

How to Measure BBT

Shake down a basal thermometer and place it at your bedside. Upon awakening turn on the bedside lamp if the room is dark, then place the thermometer snugly in your armpit. While lying in bed without any extra motion, wait for ten minutes, then record the temperature reading. Repeat this for five consecutive days.

If you are still menstruating, take your temperature beginning the second day of the menstrual flow. Menopausal/postmenopausal women and men can obtain their BBT at any time.

The role of thyroid function in breast cancer and/or prevention is controversial. This can better be understood when you realize that iodine is used by both the breast and the thyroid gland. Just as the improper metabolism or lack of iodine by the thyroid can result in goiter formation, the breast's cells can respond in a similar fashion resulting in cancer formation. However, many reasons for breast cancer appear to be related to the improper metabolism of iodine (discussed in Chapter 10). Iodine is a key element in the control of breast cell division. And whether your thyroid is hypo (low), hyper (high), or in the low-normal range, your immune system will function better if your thyroid hormones are normalized to the middle to upper range of accepted levels.

Thyroid Symptom Summary

A well-balanced thyroid function is of utmost importance to overall health. Therefore, all issues having to do with the thyroid and the various symptoms noted above should be addressed by a trained health professional.

Excess (hyperthyroidism): Racing heart, diarrhea, intolerance to heat, nervousness, irritability, and loss of bone.

Insufficiency/deficiencies (hypothyroidism): Fatigue or weakness, depression, weight gain, decrease in appetite, change in menstrual cycles, decrease in sex drive, cold intolerance (especially of the hands and feet), constipation, fuzzy memory, dry skin, headaches and muscle aches, puffiness around the eyes, hair loss, low basal body temperature (less than 97.4 degrees Fahrenheit), and brittle fingernails. There can also be a decreased efficiency of the immune system that can predispose one to cancer.

Here are the commonly used thyroid replacement hormones:

- Armour Thyroid, Nature-Thyroid (orally administered desiccated thyroid) which contain T4 and T3 as well as T2, T1, and calcitonin

- Thyrolar — a combination of T3 and T4

- Synthetic T4 — Synthroid, Levothyroid, etc.

- T3 SR (slow release)

- Synthetic T3 — Cytomel

Case Study: Safer Hormone Help

Sharon is 52 years old. Due to heavy bleeding and large fibroids, she had her uterus and ovaries removed almost four years ago. After the surgery she was placed on hormone replacement therapy. For the past 3½ years she has been taking a synthetic estrogen preparation daily and has not suffered from hot flashes, although she has experienced occasional breast tenderness, moderate weight gain, and a decreased desire to be sexually intimate with her husband. After listening to a constant barrage of media coverage portraying estrogen therapy as harmful, Sharon decided to stop taking her hormones "cold turkey." That was six months ago and now she admits her quality of life has worsened; she wakes up in the middle of the night drenched in sweat, feeling tired because of the interrupted sleep; she has more "down" than "up" moments; she must mentally reach for names that were once easy to remember; and she feels dry "down there."

Seeking relief, she was placed on antidepressants by her physician. This proved unsatisfactory. Her friend suggested an herbal preparation specially designed for menopause she had seen in a popular women's magazine. After using this botanical blend for almost a month she thought there might have been some improvement, but it turned out to be only temporary and her symptoms returned.

At our initial visit, Sharon decided to begin the FEM Centre Breast Care Program, and I tailored the program to suit her needs. This "change for life" included the use of bio-identical triest transdermal cream (see pages 138-139) instead of the synthetic oral estrogen preparation. Sharon was shown how to adjust the dose of the cream on her own to remain symptom-free. Progesterone was also added to the daily hormonal regimen even though Sharon had had a hysterectomy.

After several weeks, blood tests were obtained to evaluate her hormonal status. This delay in testing permitted her to begin the breast care program and allowed us to see the effect the triest preparation had on the level of estrogen in her blood. The laboratory results revealed that Sharon had insufficient levels of testosterone, DHEA, and thyroid; however, her estradiol level was at 29 pg/ml, well within our defined target range. Best of all, her night sweats had vanished, allowing for a more consistent sleep pattern.

Along with hormonal balancing, which included testosterone cream, DHEA, and thyroid replacement, Sharon had started the 21-day detox diet (Appendix B) and breast nutritional supplements (Chapter 10). Within four weeks her weight had dropped twelve pounds and energy levels were on the upswing. On that positive note, we decided to extend the detox diet for another six weeks.

Twelve weeks later we met once again to discuss her progress. Hormonal laboratory values for testosterone, DHEA, and thyroid were greatly improved. Her weight loss now totaled twenty-four pounds and the breast tenderness was gone. As Sharon put it, "Until now I never realized how bad I felt. It seems that the longer I follow the program, the better I seem to feel."

Melatonin

Melatonin is the body's all-natural sleep aid. At night, as our optical nerves note the fall of darkness, melatonin is produced by the pineal gland, a pea-size structure at the center of the brain. This remarkable hormone regulates our sleep/wake cycles. The secretion of melatonin is greatest between 1 and 4 a.m. When the eye registers any appreciable light, melatonin levels will drop. Not only are there daily variations but also seasonal variations: Higher levels occur in the winter (longer hours of darkness) as opposed to the summer (long days, short nights).

And why is sleep so important to good health? The body requires a certain amount of deep sleep known as rapid eye movement (REM) sleep to function properly. During REM sleep, your body enters a healing, detoxification, and rejuvenating mode both physically and mentally.

Studies have shown that chronic lack of this deep sleep can lead to mood changes, depression, physical illness, and even psychosis. Low levels of melatonin have been implicated in breast cancer, depression of the immune system, mood changes, and disturbances in the sleep/wake cycle. When the eyes are exposed to total darkness, the brain's internal clock induces the pineal gland to release melatonin, and disruption to this finely tuned system can be caused by jet lag, working night shifts, exposure to light in the early morning hours, but most often by age and the inevitable march of time.

As we get older, the amount of melatonin produced by our body diminishes (see Figure 13, page 154). Melatonin begins to decline by age 40, and by age 60, less than half is produced. The pineal gland can also be subject to calcification (especially in the elderly), so it is not just coincidence that sleep problems occur with greater frequency in midlife and beyond.

Melatonin also has another important role — in animal studies, melatonin has been shown to be a powerful, neutralizing, free-radical scavenger that can penetrate into every cell, making it one of the most potent antioxidants in the human body. These antioxidant effects are thought to enhance the thymus and protect the brain, breasts, and even the heart. (Free radicals are constantly being generated by the production of cellular energy to sustain cell function. Aging and the onset of chronic diseases such as heart disease and cancer are hastened by free radical buildup.)

Melatonin is also very important in the prevention of breast cancer. Studies have shown that women who work night shifts have a 60 percent increased risk of developing breast cancer, especially if they work between 1 and 2 a.m. Blind women, meanwhile, have a very low incidence of breast cancer. We have already noted that melatonin begins to drop after age 40 (and especially at 60), which parallels the increase in breast cancer incidence.

In addition to being a potent antioxidant, melatonin enhances the immune system, blocks estrogen from overstimulating your breast cells, starves cancer by preventing new blood vessel growth, and blocks uncontrolled breast cell division. Melatonin may prevent breast cancer as a result of its antiestrogenic properties, especially that of decreasing aromatase activity. Scientists have found that melatonin in high doses can be helpful in mimicking the tumor-killing ability of chemotherapy and radiation, while decreasing the side effects for those with certain cancers. (However, melatonin supplementation should be avoided in pregnancy and for those trying for pregnancy.)

Measurement of melatonin is best obtained using saliva samples, yet we tend to rely on symptoms such as interrupted sleep to determine the need for melatonin replacement.

Melatonin Application

Melatonin may be swallowed or dissolved under the tongue. One should opt for a slow-release melatonin. Begin at a dose of 0.5 to 1 mg thirty minutes before bedtime, and increase by 1 mg nightly until sleep is achieved. Sublingual doses begin at 0.3 mg and can be increased incrementally. The prolonged use of melatonin should include off intervals to permit your brain to sustain its own production.

Melatonin Symptom Summary

Excess: Drowsiness, low levels of sex hormones, possible increase in thyroid activity.

Deficiency: Insomnia, increased risk of breast cancer, chronic diseases of the brain, heart disease.

Cortisol (a corrosive hormone of aging)

For millions of years when a human was faced with danger, the ensuing "fight or flight" syndrome caused the adrenal glands to release cortisol, often referred to as the "stress hormone." A surge in cortisol causes a chain-reaction of almost instantaneous physiological events, culminating in the increase of one's blood sugar level so that the brain will have more glucose for energy (to fight or flee). This, in turn, causes other tissues of the body to decrease their glucose fuel requirements, and leads to the release of energy sources from fat cells for use by the muscles (again, to fight or flee). All of these energy transformations ready the individual to deal with a stressful situation or an imminent danger.

Primitive humans didn't spend much time worrying about the future or dwelling on the past, so their cortisol levels rose only in response to physical threats. Unfortunately, modern society has altered the ancient pattern of cortisol release.

Since cortisol secretion increases in response to any stress in the body, whether physical or psychological, the modern individual activates the "fight or flight" syndrome many times throughout an average day. The pressure of work, traffic jams, money, family — any one of these psychological events can trigger the release of cortisol.

When we experience a stressful psychological event, there is an outpouring of cortisol, which tends to break down protein such as that found in muscle, to provide glucose for energy. During this acute phase, a person tends to lose weight. (This is weight loss attributed to the stress of a divorce, a career change, the death of a loved one, etc.)

In a long-term state of chronic stress, a continual release of cortisol alters the physiology of the body much the same as chronic administration of prednisone. (People who are on corticosteroids such as prednisone for long periods gain weight, especially in the mid-abdomen, face, and that area around the back of one's neck that we call a buffalo hump.) By now, the receptors on cells are tired of being stimulated by the relentless release of cortisol. In fact, they do not respond to usual dosage levels, leading to a further disruption of the body's equilibrium. When receptors become resistant to cortisol, you become susceptible to infections and subsequent diseases. Your health further deteriorates. One can see a self-perpetuating downward spiral, all caused by stress and its partner, cortisol.

But cortisol serves as more than a simple response to stress. Cortisol is essential for the functioning of almost every part of the body. Cortisol has a role in the regulation of blood pressure, cardiovascular function, and the body's processing of proteins, carbohydrates, and fats. Too much or too little of this crucial hormone can also lead to many physical symptoms and disease states.

Cortisol is quite toxic to nerve cells, especially those that reside in that area of the brain responsible for memory — the hippocampus. For this reason, continued exposure to excess levels of cortisol can increase the risk for dementia and other neurological diseases.

As we age, our levels of cortisol begin to rise 25 percent above earlier levels, and a chronic excess of cortisol may have a detrimental effect on the attempt to balance hormones. A chronic increase in cortisol ultimately lowers growth hormones, thyroid hormones, and sex hormones, and contributes to lowered immune function. This certainly sets the stage for chronic diseases.

Blood levels of cortisol normally peak in the morning to provide energy throughout the day, decreasing in the evening to allow for rest. As one ages, the natural pattern changes, with peaks also occurring in the nighttime hours. This can cause you to awaken too early — instead of returning to sleep, you lie there with a racing mind.

An insufficiency in cortisol may manifest itself as fatigue that comes and goes throughout the day. Certainly fatigue after a particularly stressful event will be suggestive. There may also be an increase in allergy symptoms.

A physician should assess your cortisol levels. Not only is it important to determine whether there is a cortisol excess or insufficiency but also *when* peak levels occur during the day and evening hours. Studies show a higher risk of breast cancer, along with a greater incidence of metastasis, with an evening cortisol spike. Researchers also report that women with advanced breast cancer who have abnormal daytime levels of cortisol are more likely to die sooner than patients with normal levels of the hormone. Studies have also found that women with abnormal cortisol levels had fewer immune system cells.

Cortisol Symptom Summary

The imbalances of cortisol that we have been discussing should not be confused with medical illnesses such as Cushing's syndrome and Addison's disease. Prompt medical intervention is required for these conditions.

Excess: Cushing syndrome involves prolonged excess exposure to cortisol, which can lead to elevated blood pressure, central obesity, striae (skin stretch marks), diabetes, excess hair growth, and rounded facial features. Cushing's syndrome results from pathological causes such as brain lesions, adrenal tumors, or excessive use of steroid medications. By contrast, the excess cortisol secretion that we address in our program results from functional imbalances. Over a period of time symptoms of functional hypercortisolism can resemble those of Cushing's syndrome.

Insufficiency: Tiring easily, predisposed to hypoglycemia, susceptibility to infection, and increased allergies. Treatment consists of either adrenal support or orally administered slow-release cortisol.

Deficiency: Hypocortisol production, such as found in Addison's disease, is potentially life-threatening and requires medical intervention.

Insulin

A hormone made in the pancreas, insulin provides your body with the means to control blood sugar so that the brain, heart, and every cell will have an adequate energy supply. Insulin is one of those crucial hormones that affect every other aspect of health, including the ability to balance the other hormones discussed in this chapter. The key to healthy aging starts with proper control of insulin, which in turn promotes the proper balancing of other hormones.

By binding to specific cell receptors, insulin allows glucose (the all-important fuel that enables cell machinery to function) to enter the cell from the bloodstream.

At its worst, insulin can initiate inflammatory conditions that can clog the arteries of the heart, lead to an impaired immune system, and even provide the means for uncontrolled cellular division (breast cancer).

As we age, our cells become resistant to insulin. Reacting to this resistance, the pancreas releases even larger amounts. The resulting excess insulin eventually causes an overabsorption of sugar into the cell, reducing levels of blood sugar (a condition called hypoglycemia).

Some of us can see the effects of insulin imbalance just by standing naked in front of a mirror. If you have a predominant midsection that gives your body the form of an apple, you've experienced an accumulation of fat cells based on insulin resistance.

If there is too little insulin, levels of sugar will rise in the blood and can become life-threatening. This is known as insulin-dependent diabetes.

Cancer cells can survive only with a steady diet of sugar, which is why they have almost one-hundred times the insulin receptors of normal cells. Women who have had breast cancer and have abnormally elevated insulin levels when fasting have a tenfold higher chance of metastasis.

An epidemic of insulin dysfunction is now sweeping our society, including our children. This "metabolic syndrome" is manifested by lack of control of insulin in response to the food that we eat and is associated with an increased risk of heart disease, high blood pressure, abnormal cholesterol levels, and diabetes. Polycystic ovary syndrome, characterized by irregular menses, high blood pressure, and increased hair growth, is another manifestation of insulin imbalance.

Diet is the primary controller of insulin levels. Basically, following a "no wheat, no sweets" eating plan as described in Chapter 7, will keep insulin levels in check.

Human Growth Hormone (HGH)

Human growth hormone, produced by the pituitary gland in the brain, is considered by some to be the hormone of youthfulness, but it is not without controversy. HGH is also known as somatotrophin.

Upon release from the brain, HGH acts primarily on two tissues: fat cells and the liver. Binding to fat cells results in the release of fat, which provides the energy to build and restore muscle and organ tissue. Binding to liver cells results in the production of insulin-like Growth Factor 1 (IGF-1), which promotes tissue growth. Since HGH is released in a pulsating manner and lasts only five to six minutes in the blood, IGF-1, which lasts twelve to fifteen hours, is used as an indirect measure of HGH.

HGH controls the body's production of proteins, carbohydrates, electrolytes, and fat metabolism. HGH helps your organs such as the heart, brain, muscle, and lungs to regenerate, reducing some biological aspects of aging.

Our highest levels occur when we are young, and they begin to fall 10 to 15 percent per decade. By age sixty, we have less than half of what we started with (Figure 13, page 154). Aging of the body is manifested by a slowing of metabolism with an increase in fat (as much as 50 percent), along with a decline in muscle or lean weight (as much as 30 percent).

As with other hormones (especially insulin), your cells also develop a resistance to HGH. Even though you still make HGH at age sixty, your cells do not respond as they did at age twenty.

And like melatonin, secretion generally occurs between 1 and 4 a.m., allowing your body to repair itself while you sleep. This melatonin/sleep/HGH connection clearly illustrates how balancing one hormone can help balance others.

Current medical uses include the treatment of children determined to have short stature. HGH has also been shown to lengthen life span in people with medical deficiencies in the pituitary gland. Some studies indicate improved muscle strength, higher energy levels, improved skin elasticity, improved memory, and resistance to disease. Studies have shown that HGH can play a role in decreasing the percentage of body fat; increasing bone mass; reversing neurological degeneration; improving the function of the immune system and organs such as the heart, kidneys, and lungs; and enhancing skin thickness, tone, and elasticity, as well as exercise performance, sex drive, and operation of the endocrine glands.

Human growth hormone deficiency is characterized by a decrease in muscle mass, an increase in the fat around the mid-section, a decrease in exercise capacity, bone loss, abnormal cholesterol levels, and a decreased sense of well-being.

There are natural ways to increase HGH. Enhancing and regulating sleep habits allows for the normal release of HGH (almost 75 percent of HGH is released at night while in the stages of deep sleep). A proper diet can help, along with the use of anaerobic exercise, especially resistance training. However, a formal program to increase and/or balance HGH should be carried out with a doctor's supervision.

Concerns have been expressed as to a relationship between cancer and human growth hormone. While most studies have been on animals, we can look at certain syndromes such as acromegaly, which involves the abnormally elevated secretion of HGH, and children of short stature who have been given HGH injections. Investigators have not clearly defined any increase in cancer occurrence in people with acromegaly, nor have children who have undergone HGH injections for years been reported to have an increase in cancer. Quite the contrary: HGH has been shown to increase cellular immunity, regenerate the thymus, inhibit the spread of cancer in animals, and improve the quality of life in terminal cancer patients.

It is the growth factors such as IGF-1 that seem to have a role in certain cancers. These cancers produce their own IGF-1 in order to sustain uncontrolled growth. IGF-1 promotes cell growth and inhibits programmed cell death while decreasing the amount of time a cell needs to divide. These are all potential malignant characteristics if not controlled and balanced properly.

The balancer of IGF-1 is its binding protein, IGFBP-3. This particular binding protein determines the amount of free IGF-1 available to the cells, while also inhibiting cell division and slowing the cell division cycle.

IGFBP-3 is the cancer-fighting protein that helps to control any tumor-causing effects of IGF-1. Interesting enough, the administration of HGH increases levels of IGFBP-3.

Women who are not taking HGH replacement therapy but exhibit elevated IGF-1 levels have been found to be at risk for cancers such as breast cancer. These levels are higher than those that should be attempted to achieve anti-aging effects. If you have such levels, then you are not a candidate for HGH. Based only on theoretical considerations, current recommendations advise against using HGH replacement if you have had cancer at all.

HGH Administration

Dosage: HGH replacement is accomplished using daily injections (usually six days on and one day off). The molecule is too large to pass through the digestive system membranes. Many so-called HGH supplements that are sold are what we term "secretogogues." These products are designed to enhance the release of HGH and are not HGH itself. In our experience, they achieve a modest 40 percent increase in HGH levels, which is not adequate for most women.

CHAPTER 10

Breast Care Nutrients

Three key goals of the FEM Centre Breast Care Program are to keep estrogen at a safe level within the breast cells, to reduce the bad forms of estrogen and encourage the good forms, and control breast cell division.

As noted in Chapter 4, there are three kinds of estrogen metabolites: the beneficial form, 2-hydroxy, and the potentially harmful types, 4-hydroxy and 16alpha-hydroxy. You will also remember that because fat cells and the breast manufacture their own estrogen, it is not necessarily the estrogen you take, but the estrogen you make that is the crucial factor in breast health.

Research shows that certain nutritional supplements are capable of inhibiting the initiation and growth of breast cancer. Based on these studies, and combined with clinical experience at the FEM Centre, I've developed a combination of nutrients designed to promote breast health. Figure 14 shows the general effects of several of these nutrients on estrogen levels. Calcium D-glucarate reduces the amount of estrogen available for conversion to estradiol in the breast cell, while red wine extract inhibits the enzyme (aromatase) responsible for estradiol production. The nutrients contained in our recommended multivitamin, along with diindolylmethane (DIMN), folinic acid, and folic acid, are meant to help metabolize estradiol in the breast cell by favoring the formation of the downstream methylated metabolite of 2-hydroxyestrogen (2-methoxyestrogen).

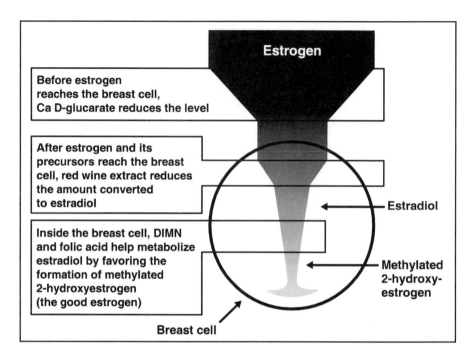

Figure 14. The effects breast care nutrients have on estrogen.

A Four-Component Breast Care Supplement Program

Although intended to promote breast health, the following nutritional components also may be used in a wellness program for the brain, heart, and bones.

The components of the Breast Care Supplement Program are:

- An iodine supplement

- An omega-3 fatty acids supplement (fish oil)

- A daily multivitamin

- A combination of diindolylmethane (DIMN), red wine extract, and calcium D-glucarate. (BreastSecure is a combination of these three supplements in a single product. Although there are several similar products on the market, we have found this particular one to be superior due to its enhanced absorption capabilities.) *Note: See Appendix E for a source for BreastSecure.*

Iodine

Almost ten years ago Dr. Jonathan Wright, an astute clinician, introduced me to the importance of iodine in relation to breast health. Since then I have used his protocol on numerous occasions to effectively dissolve fibrocystic changes of the breast.

One clue to iodine's relation to breast health can be found in world populations that have a low incidence of cancer, such as Japan. Breast, ovarian, and uterine cancer in Japanese women is less prevalent than in women in the United States. This may be related to the fact the average Japanese diet contains not only an abundance of fish (see omega-3 fatty acids, later in this chapter) but also seaweed, which is a great source of iodine. In fact, the average intake of iodine daily by a Japanese woman is 13.8 mg — almost one hundred times the Recommended Daily Allowance (RDA) dose. Iodine is a mineral that is vital to breast health and the proper functioning of the thyroid gland. Iodine helps cells return to normal and aids in apoptosis, or programmed cell death. (This is the opposite of cancer, where cells ignore the body's natural apoptosis and continue to propagate out of control.)

Researchers in Canada have reported using an iodine preparation in more than 3,000 women who lived in the Ontario area for a total of 10,000 woman years. The incidence of breast cancer for these 3,000 women was 0.00079 per woman year, while the overall incidence for women in the same age bracket who did not take the iodine preparation was twice that rate, at 0.00164.

Case Study: Fibrocystic Breasts and Iodine

Kathy is 43 years old and for years has had painful cystic breasts. At times they could be so tender that even getting dressed was next to impossible. She had suffered from infertility whose cause was most likely related to the endometriosis — diagnosed in her late twenties. Even though she avoided caffeine and often used vitamin E, she frequently had to return to the radiologist for follow-up mammograms to ensure that her cystic breasts' densely clustered nodules had not developed signs indicating possible malignant changes. Once again, the mammogram report read "very dense tissue with multiple cystic complexes and oval nodular densities throughout each breast." Although listed as probably benign, the recommendation, as so many times before, was to return in six months for a repeat mammogram.

At my suggestion, she began a daily regimen of 25 mg of a formulated iodine supplement consisting of both iodide and molecular iodine. Within two months the breast pain began to subside and after five months was completely absent. Her next mammogram report revealed "marked improvements" in fibrocystic features with a considerable decrease in tissue density and a decline in the number and size of nodules. The radiologist was so impressed that he even asked her what she had done differently.

While fibrocystic nodules may not be premalignant, it is the underlying process of prolonged estrogen over-stimulation to the breast cell that is worrisome. Women with fibrocystic changes have twice the risk of breast cancer. Iodine has been shown to work by interrupting excessive division at the cellular level, which can result in shrinkage of fibrocystic breast nodules.

Using both subjective evaluation (freedom from pain) and objective evaluation (resolution of fibrosis as documented by mammograms), Ghent and Eskin reported in the 1993 *Canadian Journal of Surgery* that almost 74 percent of women with documented fibrocystic breast disease experienced clinical improvement after iodine treatment.

Studies done by Doctors Abraham and Derry have determined that the breasts need approximately 5 mg of iodine daily while the thyroid needs 2 to 3 mg iodide daily.

Iodine also helps with the metabolization of estrogen, decreasing 16alpha-hydroxy, that form of estrogen mentioned earlier as one of the main foes in the battle against breast cancer.

After the thyroid, the breast is the second-most important reservoir for iodine. The reason for this is that the breast provides a new-born baby with its only source of iodine, which is crucial for early neurological development and thyroid maintenance.

Food sources of iodine include kelp, seaweed, iodized salt, and milk. (Iodine is used to sterilize cow udders, so some iodine can end up in the milk supply). Unfortunately American diets are lacking in sufficient iodine as documented in the National Health and Nutrition Survey. This study reported a 50 percent decline in dietary iodine intake over the last thirty years.

Iodine tends to attach to receptors that are located throughout the body. If enough iodine is present to occupy these receptors, any excess will be excreted into the urine. Using this concept, Drs. Abraham and Flechas developed an iodine-loading test that works by administering a standard dose of iodine in tablet form and subsequently measuring the amount of iodine excreted in the urine over the next 24 hours. (See Appendix E for the source for this test.) An iodine-sufficient state is present when 90 percent of the iodine ingested is recovered in the urine.

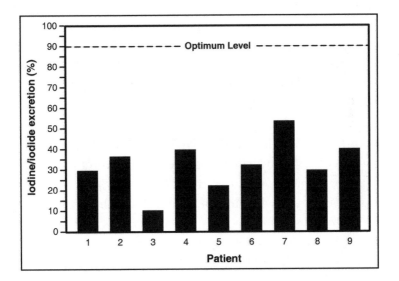

Figure 15. Results of iodine loading tests on nine consecutive breast cancer patients.

Figure 15 depicts the results of the iodine-loading tests performed on nine consecutive breast cancer patients who were seen at the FEM Centre. The uniformly low iodine levels reinforce the need for adequate supplementation.

Inadequate intake of iodine may not be the only reason for lowered iodine reserves. Iodine is listed in the table of periodic elements as a halogen. Bromine, chlorine, and fluorine are also halogens. These elements are commonly found in our environment and have similar atomic structures that permit them to be substitutes for one another. An atom of bromine can potentially displace an atom of iodine from its receptor.

Dr. Brownstein and co-investigators have proposed that the increased ingestion of halogens, especially bromine, may be implicated in the rise of breast cancer rates. He compared bromine levels in eight women with breast cancer to eight women with no history of breast cancer. Those women with breast cancer had statistically higher levels of bromine.

Bromine can be found in carbonated drinks, pesticides, over-the-counter medications, and bakery products, which may explain why Americans are an iodine-deficient population.

There is both misunderstanding and controversy surrounding iodine supplementation. Much of this relates to the organic iodine preparations that do not provide the form of iodine that our breast care program utilizes. The iodine preparations we use are inorganic and should not be confused with those used in pharmaceutical brands. (Several references listed in the bibliography further explain the role of inorganic iodine in your overall health.)

For those women who do not ingest daily amounts of seaweed comparable to that of the Japanese (brown and red seaweeds such as kombu and focus), we make use of the ideal form of iodine supplementation — Lugol's solution. Lugol's solution is a combination of iodine and iodide. This is an important combination, since iodine is a molecular form and works in the breast whereas iodide (the attachment of sodium or potassium to iodine) works in the thyroid. Together, they contribute to improved thyroid function and breast health. This combination is available in tablet form, but requires a physician to monitor iodine levels and thyroid function.

Since iodine is an essential element for thyroid hormone function (thyroxine has 4 iodine atoms while triiodothyronine has 3), it is very unlikely that one has an allergy to inorganic iodine. (Allergies to shellfish or the iodine dye used in medical imaging do not necessarily indicate allergies to inorganic iodine, but caution is always advisable.)

Omega-3 Fatty Acids (Fish Oil)
(EPA +DHA = 1.5 to 3 grams)

Omega-3 fatty acids cannot be made by the human body and must be derived from the diet. Plants such as algae manufacture omega-3s that, when ingested, accumulate in animals, especially fish. Deep, cold-water fish have high levels of omega-3 fatty acids that are used to insulate them from the frigid temperatures of the water in which they swim.

There are two types of omega-3 fatty acids found in fish oil that are very beneficial to the breast — EPA (eicosapentaenoic acid) and DHA (docosahexaenoic acid). A different type of omega-3 — alpha linolenic acid — is found in flaxseed, which we discussed in Chapter 3.

EPA and DHA have positive effects on almost every aspect of health, including the heart, blood, bones, breasts, and brain. These omega-3s help cells retain their fluidity, which means they're better able to communicate with neighboring cells. This is important because cancerous cells often don't recognize when to stop dividing, meaning they continue to grow, multiply, and trespass onto other cells' territories.

Omega-3s also act as anti-inflammatory agents (in proper doses they are as effective as a non-steroidal anti-inflammatory drugs and are much safer). Chronic inflammation is a problem underlying many of the discomforts and diseases related to aging, and may play an important role in encouraging or laying the foundation for cancer.

Omega-3 fatty acids also modulate the breakdown of estrogens. EPA causes 16alpha-hydroxyestrogen to decrease while increasing the good 2-hydroxyestrogen. DHA decreases the number of estrogen receptors on ER+ breast cancer cells, slowing their growth.

Ideally, omega-3 fatty acids are obtained from fish, but the amounts can vary and there is the additional problem in fish of mercury and other heavy metal contamination. For this reason, a high quality fish oil supplement that has undergone rigorous molecular distillation to remove heavy metals is recommended. (Be sure and find out the metal content of the fish oil you plan to use.)

Fish oil comes in soft gel capsules or liquid form. The strength of the capsules can be found by adding the listed amount of EPA and DHA that is contained in each capsule. This number will be different from the total amount of fat listed for the capsule.

Our recommended dosage is calculated to provide your body with the quantity and ratio of EPA and DHA we believe is necessary for preventive purposes. Should you be experiencing arthritis, heart disease, or neurological disease, higher doses may be required. However, taking higher doses of omega-3 daily for prevention may not be beneficial in the long term. Our laboratory studies show that you *can* take too much omega-3, resulting in deficiencies of omega-6 fatty acids. (The optimal consumption ratio of omega-6 to omega-3 is about 4 to 1.)

Multivitamin Supplement

A good multivitamin is essential to overall health, and is especially important in the FEM Centre Breast Care Program. Most of the once-a-day vitamins available to consumers lack sufficient amounts of the key ingredients we believe are needed to optimize their preventive effects.

Some sixty years ago the FDA established Minimum Daily Requirements (MDR) for vitamins and minerals. These values were set to encourage the prevention of goiters. Since then, the FDA has changed the minimum daily requirement standard to the Recommended Daily Allowance (RDA) of vitamins and minerals. This was done to address the problem of over-consumption of these supplements — a side effect of the previous standard. It is important to understand, however, that neither the MDR values of old or the current RDA values address the question of the levels of vitamins and minerals necessary for the prevention of disease, especially relative to the latest scientific research concerning breast health.

A good multivitamin supplement should contain vitamins, minerals, and important antioxidants. The list on the following page contains the suggested ingredients that should be present in a good daily multivitamin and mineral supplement.

The role of antioxidants has frequently been challenged, especially in traditional medical circles. Antioxidants function as biologic sponges soaking up DNA-damaging free radicals, which are being continuously generated by the body. Epidemiological studies clearly show that a high intake of antioxidant-rich foods decreases the risk of cancer and that vitamin C and E reduce the incidence of breast cancer recurrence.

An antioxidant should not be used as a stand-alone or single agent; instead a combination produces the healthiest results, especially when the antioxidants are in the form of whole foods. Traditional medicine attempts to evaluate the effectiveness of a single antioxidant in much the same way as a pharmaceutical drug would be tested. For instance, studies that make use of only vitamin E ignore the fact that the action of vitamin E depends upon other antioxidants, namely vitamin C. Also, there are different forms of vitamin E, each of which has an important antioxidant role. The majority of traditional medicine studies have used only the alpha form of vitamin E, which I believe is incorrect.

Another word of caution: Many studies are conducted using either isolated cell cultures (*in vitro*) or special types of laboratory animals. The results of these tests may or may not reflect the *in vivo* conditions found in the human body.

Note: The following recommended vitamins and minerals should be taken under supervision of a physician.

Recommended Amounts of Key Vitamins and Minerals:
Dosage note: mg = milligrams
mcg = micrograms
IU = International Units

- Vitamin A — 5000 to 10,000 IU

- Vitamin C — 500 to 1,000 mg

- Vitamin D3 — 800 to 1,000 IU

- Vitamin E — 400 to 800 IU as mixed tocopherols (Vitamin E helps in treatment and prevention of fibrocystic changes that occur in the breast.)

- Thiamine — 75 mg

- Riboflavin (vitamin B2) — 75 mg

- Niacin — 75 mg

- Vitamin B6 — more than 50 mg

- Folic acid — 800 mcg

- Vitamin B12 — 150 mcg (in the form of methylcobalamin, which is better absorbed by the brain)

- Biotin — 75 mcg

- Pantothenic acid — 100 mg

- Calcium — approximately 250 mg (as hydroxyapatite)

- Iodine — (see page 176)

- Magnesium — 500 mg (2 to 1 ratio of magnesium to calcium)

- Zinc — 30 mg

- Selenium — 200 to 400 mcg

- Copper — 2 mg

- Manganese — 5 mg

- Chromium — 200 mcg

- Molybdenum — 50 mcg

- Potassium — 99 mg

- Boron — 2 mg to 4 mg (Boron is essential for bone health and also helps balance hormones.)

Note: Magnesium, zinc, selenium, copper, manganese, chromium, and molybdenum are best absorbed as chelates.

Vitamin D is of particular importance in maintaining breast health, promoting bone integrity, and balancing the immune system. Sunlight activates a special type of cholesterol molecule located in the skin to form vitamin D, which acts more like a hormone than a vitamin.

I recommend not only daily vitamin D supplementation, but also exposure to midday sunlight for five to ten minutes, three times weekly. The vitamin D that is ingested or created by your body is then transformed into the biologically active form in the liver and kidneys. Activated vitamin D works at the DNA level of the breast cell to initiate programmed cell death, thus preventing uncontrolled cell division (cancer).

I recommend using vitamin D3 (cholecalciferol) to achieve blood levels that fall in the upper normal range. After testing hundreds of women, less than 10 percent have had optimal levels of vitamin D3. Multivitamins generally will not contain amounts of vitamin D3 (1,000 to 5,000 IU and higher) needed to raise blood levels. However, the dose must be individualized according to your blood levels.

Because vitamin D appears to influence cancer risk, we advise that blood levels be checked on a regular basis. Studies have shown that the farther away one moves from the equator (and its more intense sunlight), the higher the prevalence of breast and prostate cancer. Women who have mutations in their vitamin D receptor may have double the risk for breast cancer.

Folic acid is a B-complex vitamin found in dark leafy green vegetables, beans, fruits, whole grains, and some fortified breakfast cereals. Along with vitamin B6 and vitamin B12, folic acid prevents the DNA within the breast cell from turning cancerous by a process called methylation. (Methylation is the placement of a methyl group — CH_3 — at the end of a molecule. This is analogous to placing a period at the end of a sentence. Uncontrolled cell division stops, and the 2-hydroxyestrogens are armed to kill cancer cells, while the 4-hydroxyestrogens are inactivated and no longer able to harm breast cell DNA.)

Almost 30 percent of the population cannot methylate properly as a result of the inborn genetic variations of two enzymes methylenetetrahydrofolate reductase (MTHFR) and catechol-O-methyltransferase (COMT). This means that higher levels of folic acid are required in their diet.

Special genomic testing is available to help identify women who are at risk for these genetic coding problems. Insufficient activity of the enzyme MTHFR can elevate blood levels of homocysteine. We recommend checking homocysteine to detect methylation efficiency. Suggested levels should be 6 to 7μmol/L. Increases in homocysteine are frequently mirrored by the elevation of other inflammation parameters such as high-sensitivity C-reactive protein. COMT also participates in the methylation process by converting 2-hydroxyestrogens to the breast cancer-killing 2-methoxyestrogens while deactivating the cancer causing 4-hydroxyestrogens. A decrease in COMT activity could create a hostile hormonal environment within the breast cell.

DNA research has shown that the risk of breast cancer may increase in those women with lower levels of folic acid, and there is plenty of data to suggest that folic acid may reduce the risk of many other types of cancer, especially colon cancer. A Harvard study published in the *Annals of Internal Medicine* reported that women with a high intake of folic acid were 75 percent less likely to get colon cancer than those with a lower intake. Low levels of folic acid have been associated with higher rates of birth defects (e.g., spina bifida and anencephaly), heart disease and even Alzheimer's.

Dr. W. Van Niekerk made the first studies noting a connection between cancer and folic acid in the 1960s. His study found several similarities between cells from the cervix in women who were deficient in folic acid and cervical cells showing early signs of cancer. In the 1980s, a study at the University of Alabama suggested a connection between folic acid and abnormal cells in the cervix. Recently, studies have shown that cervical cancer was more likely to develop in women with lower levels of folic acid.

During the last few years, researchers have accumulated data to show a connection between low levels of folic acid and cancer of the breast, lung, esophagus, and stomach.

Few people eat enough leafy green vegetables to produce the optimum amount of folic acid, so a nutritional supplement is a key component in our breast care program.

Selenium is an important trace element whose insufficiency is also common in the U.S. population. Derived from the food you eat, the inadequate amounts available in the American diet are due to poor crop rotation practices that leach the element out of the soil. In addition, heavy metals such as arsenic have been shown to interfere with selenium.

Studies show that adequate amounts of selenium are required for the thyroid to effectively make use of iodine. The anti-cancer effects of selenium, including apoptosis, have been well-documented by studies that have appeared in numerous publications.

Case Study: It's the Hormone You Make

At age 29, Gail noticed a lemon-size mass in her right breast. She underwent a biopsy, which revealed a diagnosis of ER+ ductal cell breast cancer. Subsequently a right-side mastectomy was performed.

Seeing Gail for the first time almost four years later, I suggested that she have a hormonal profile that measured her estrogen metabolites, namely 2-hydroxyestrone and 16alpha-hydroxyestrone. (Studies by Bradlow and associates have shown an increased risk of premenopausal breast cancer in those women with depressed 2-hydroxyestrogen:16alpha-hydroxyestrogen ratios — 2-hydroxyestrogens are capable of killing breast cancer cells while the 16alpha-hydroxyestrogens can increase tumor growth.) It was time to be proactive and begin the FEM Center Breast Care Program.

Gail's initial 2-hydroxyestrogen levels were on the low side, at 126 pg/ml, while her 16alpha-hydroxy levels were moderately elevated at 326 pg/ml. Her ratio of 2-hydroxyestrogen:16alpha-hydroxyestrogen was 0.39 — too low, especially for a breast cancer survivor. I prefer a ratio of 0.9 or greater.

She was subsequently placed on a daily dose of BreastSecure, which uses an enhanced-delivery form of DIMN, calcium D-glucarate, and red wine extract. Three weeks later I repeated her lab work and found that her 2-hydroxyestrone was at 216 pg/ml, while her 16alpha-hydroxy levels had dropped to 228 pg/ml. This represented a new ratio of 0.95 — a vast improvement. With an elevation of the 2-hydroxyestrogens she had increased her body's ability to fight recurrent breast cancer while also lowering the tumor-forming 16alpha-hydroxy.

Gail's breast cancer had nothing to do with estrogen replacement and illustrates once again that it is the hormones your body makes, not those you take, that deserve the most concern.

BreastSecure

Diindolylmethane, calcium D-glucarate, and red wine extract are essential ingredients used in our breast care program. Taken individually or in combination, these nutritional supplements have beneficial specialized chemotherapeutic actions on the breasts. Whether one decides to be on hormonal therapy or to not use hormones at all, I suggest the lifelong use of these supplements.

For maximum absorption and convenience I recommend Breast-Secure, which is a dietary supplement featuring an enhanced delivery system for DIMN, red wine extract, and calcium D-glucarate. The suggested dose is one to two capsules daily.

DIMN (Diindolylmethane)
(75 to 100 milligrams)

As mentioned earlier, estradiol (one of the three forms of estrogen) is converted into 2-hydroxy, 4-hydroxy, and 16alpha-hydroxy. DIMN increases estrogen conversion to the healthier 2-hydroxy while discouraging the production of the potentially harmful 4-hydroxy and 16alpha-hydroxy.

DIMN is a natural derivative of certain vegetables that are known as *cruciferous*. Cruciferous vegetables (cabbage, broccoli, cauliflower, Brussels sprouts, etc.) contain nutrients that have remarkable properties that aid in the prevention of cancer. One of these ingredients is indole-3-carbinol. In the stomach's acidic environment, under optimal conditions, indole-3-carbinol is broken down into DIMN, which must be absorbed across the intestinal wall to reach the bloodstream and contribute its positive effects. Unfortunately, we are unable to consume sufficient amounts of these vegetables to maximize the benefits of DIMN. (It would take several pounds of broccoli daily to obtain an effective level of DIMN. It is also poorly absorbed, which is why one needs an enhanced-absorption delivery system to achieve effective levels in the blood.)

DIMN is delivered to various tissues in the body and bathes the cells there, promoting the formation of 2-hydroxyestrogen and reducing the creation of 4-hydroxyestrogen and 16alpha-hydroxyestrogen. DIMN enters the breast cell and binds to a special receptor — the aryl hydrocarbon receptor. This chemical reaction has two protective effects: 1) the resulting complex (DIMN-ARYL) blocks cell division both in estrogen receptor positive (ER+) and estrogen receptor negative (ER-) tumors, and 2) it activates an enzyme, CYP1A1, which increases the production of breast cancer killing 2-hydroxyestrogens.

Currently, there is a debate about whether it is better to use indole-3-carbinol or DIMN. Our clinical experience, a review of the medical literature, and personal conversations with researchers who have investigated the relationship of estrogen metabolites to breast cancer indicate that DIMN is the superior ingredient. Plus, research has revealed that the protective role of DIMN is not just limited to the breast but also extends to other hormonally sensitive tissues like the prostate, the uterus, and even the ovaries.

Indole-3-carbinol conversion to DIMN requires an acidic environment in the stomach; however, adequate stomach acidity is a problem for many women in midlife. Also, studies reveal that DIMN is present only in cells initially incubated with indole-3-carbinol. Indole-3-carbinol may metabolize into the potential carcinogen-producing indolocarbazole.

Hormonal studies at the FEM Centre confirm an almost 75 percent increase in 2-hydroxyestrogens using the enhanced delivery system for DIMN contained in BreastSecure.

After ingesting DIMN, your urine may turn amber. Don't panic. This indicates adequate absorption but it also means you need to drink more water. Patients should also note that because DIMN controls the breakdown of estrogen, there are some theoretical concerns that it may decrease the effectiveness of birth control pills, and it is probably a good idea to avoid using DIMN during pregnancy.

Red Wine Extract
(200 to 400 milligrams. Does not contain potentially allergenic sulfites and tannins that are found in red wine.)

Nature has provided us with a powerful tool grown in the soil and nourished by the sun and the rain — grapes used in the making of red wine. Studies have shown that moderate consumption of red wine (but not white) has been linked to a decrease in breast density, and a reduction in risk for cancer and heart disease. Red wine also provides a host of other benefits. These studies inspired researchers to isolate the positive components of red wine, and the result of that research is red wine extract.

Red wine extract is an alcohol-free, whole food supplement that consists of a concentrated blend of red grape skins and seeds. This combination is a rich source of breast-friendly compounds that include resveratrol, quercitin, and rutin — compounds synthesized by a grapevine in response to injury or to ward off fungal attacks.

Red wine extract contains a combination of powerful anti-oxidants and estrogen modulators that protect against endometriosis, fibroids, and breast cancer. Red wine extract not only encourages breast health, but it also protects the brain, heart, and bones, and appears to reduce dementia in the elderly. Resveratrol is a key component, and has many positive qualities:

- Reduces the amount of estrogen available for conversion to estrogen metabolites (the "usual suspects" in the formation of breast cancer)

- Chelates (removes/detoxifies) copper

- Inhibits production of LDL, the plaque-promoting cholesterol

- Decreases abnormal blood platelet clumping

- Has anti-inflammatory properties

- Has many anti-cancer activities

Red wine extract also contains ingredients, known as procyanidins, which act as powerful inhibitors of the enzyme aromatase. Restricting aromatase prevents the excessive production of estradiol within the breast cell, which, as you know by now, is one of the main goals of our breast care program. Absorption of red wine extract has been attributed to the alcohol in wine, but lab data reveal that the same enhanced delivery system for DIMN also works for red wine extract. BreastSecure incorporates both of these supplements without the need for alcohol.

Improved outcomes in estrogen receptor positive (ER+) breast cancer have been noted using pharmaceutical aromatase inhibitors: Arimidex, Femara, and Aromasin. Animal studies performed by Dr. Eng have demonstrated that the aromatase-inhibiting properties of red wine extract are comparable to that of the pharmaceutical drug Femara. (Other supplements have been touted as aromatase inhibitors — such as chyrsin, naringenin, and apigenin — but these have been shown to be effective only in test tubes and not in humans.)

Calcium D-Glucarate (the "Toxic Avenger")
200 to 400 milligrams.

Studies show that high levels of the enzyme beta-glucuronidase have been found at breast tumor sites. This enzyme reduces the body's ability to detoxify and eliminate excessive estrogen, which can contribute to the risk for breast cancer.

Glucarate blocks this unwanted enzymatic reaction by up to 50 percent, thereby lowering excess estrogen levels by some 25 percent, according to some studies. It also keeps the body from reabsorbing estrogen that's marked for excretion via the intestines.

Found in apples, Brussels sprouts, broccoli, cabbage, and lettuce, glucarate is a naturally occurring substance that supports important detoxification pathways in the body, but glucarate's main importance to breast health lies in its ability to be metabolized into a natural inhibitor of beta-glucuronidase.

Calcium D-glucarate is the orally administered, sustained-release form of glucarate. It was developed and patented by M. D. Anderson Cancer Center in Houston, Texas. Calcium D-glucarate allows glucarate to circulate longer in the bloodstream in order to bathe sensitive tissues.

In more than twenty studies using animals, it has been shown to significantly reduce breast cancer formation and mammary tumor volume. Research also indicates that glucarate works synergistically with tamoxifen. In animal subjects, cancers such as prostate, lung, liver, and colon have been shown to decrease as well.

Other Supplements

There certainly are other supplements, although not mentioned in the nutritional recommendations above, which have been shown to possibly play a role in breast cancer treatment. For example, isolated reports have indicted that approximately 390 mg doses of CoQ-10 daily have resulted in breast cancer remissions, but this remains to be confirmed by subsequent studies.

I have listed only those nutrients that were included in our postmenopausal patients who were followed for almost six years and were found to have a markedly reduced incidence of breast cancer.

A prevention program must be both effective and easy to follow on a long-term basis. The FEM Centre Breast Care Program is designed primarily for the prevention of breast cancer but also serves as a foundation for aggressive treatment. Modification of our recommendations depends upon thermographic findings that indicate persistent abnormalities, mammographic abnormalities, and the presence of breast cancer in a patient.

CHAPTER 11

Mammograms/Thermograms:
The Warning Signs and
Early Detection of Breast Cancer

Screening is not the same as prevention. Screening is used to detect cancer early, whereas prevention is a lifelong series of choices
that encourage breast health. Both are vital components of our overall breast care program.

Since, at present, prevention programs are not 100 percent effective, periodic breast screening is necessary to improve the chances of
detecting breast cancer at the earliest stage. I recommend what I call
the "breast surveillance triad" consisting of: 1) frequent breast self-
exams, 2) a routine exam by a health practitioner, and 3) a periodic
breast screening using current imaging techniques which include a
combination of the thermogram and mammogram. Obviously, early
cancer detection and treatment greatly improves the outcome and
can increase the possibility of permanent remission.

Breast Self-Examination (BSE)

All too often a woman is the first to notice a lump in her breast,
making the breast self-exam very important. On numerous occasions
women have remarked that they do not perform self-examination
because of lumpy breasts. To these women I respond that self-
examination has already proved its worth by detecting their fibrocystic changes (lumpy breasts), thus reinforcing the need for imme-
diate implementation of the FEM Centre's Breast Care Program.

Even with chronic breast irregularities, the value of self-
examination lies in the fact that it alerts one to the appearance of

new lumps that, if persistent, require medical follow-up. Self-examination serves the roles of detection, identification of breast masses that may be cancerous, and prevention, by detecting conditions such as fibrocystic changes.

Timing of the breast self-exam is important. If you are still menstruating, wait until the end of your flow before self-examination. At this time hormones such as estrogen are less likely to influence breast tissue, while the initial burst of progesterone following ovulation has subsided allowing the breast tissue to be at rest. It is not uncommon to palpate cysts and experience breast tenderness after ovulation. By the end of your flow these resolve, permitting breast self-examination.

If your flows have ceased then I suggest a self-examination on a monthly basis.

How to Perform Breast Self-Examination

Note: Beginning in your twenties you should become aware of how your breasts normally feel so you will be able to detect any changes.

Begin by standing in front of a mirror with your shoulders straight and your arms by your hips. Look at your breast and note any changes in their usual size, shape, or color. Especially look for dimpling, puckering or bulging of the skin. Examine the nipple for redness, crusting, or soreness. Gently squeeze each nipple and check for a discharge (if blood-tinged, notify your physician). Raise your arms and again look for any the changes.

Lie down and place your right arm behind your head. The exam is done while lying down, and not standing up, because when lying down the breast tissue spreads evenly over the chest wall and it is as thin as possible, making it much easier to feel all of it.

Use the finger pads of the three middle fingers on your left hand to feel for lumps in the right breast. Use the finger pads your right hand to feel for lumps in the left breast. Use overlapping dime-sized circular motions of the finger pads to feel the breast tissue.

Use three different levels of pressure to feel all the breast tissue. Light pressure is needed to feel the tissue closest to the skin; medium pressure to feel a little deeper; and firm pressure to feel the tissue closest to the chest and ribs. A firm ridge in the lower curve of each breast is normal. If you're not sure how hard to press, talk with your doctor or nurse. Use each pressure level to feel the breast tissue before moving on to the next spot.

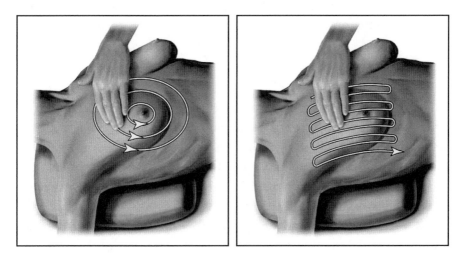

Figure 16. Breast self-exam — left, using a circular motion; right, using a vertical, up-down motion.

Move around the breast in an up-and-down pattern starting at the middle of the chest bone (sternum or breastbone) and moving across the breast to an imaginary line drawn straight down your side from the underarm. Be sure to check the entire breast area going down until you feel only ribs and up to the neck or collar bone (clavicle).

There is some evidence to suggest that the up-and-down pattern (sometimes called the vertical pattern) is the most effective pattern for covering the entire breast and not missing any breast tissue. Repeat the exam on your left breast, using the finger pads of the right hand.

Examine each underarm while sitting up or standing and with your arm only slightly raised so you can easily feel in this area. Raising your arm straight up tightens the tissue in this area and makes it very difficult to examine. Remember, if you find any changes, see your doctor right away.

Current imaging techniques used for detecting breast cancer include mammograms, ultrasound, MRI, and thermography. Newer technologies such as dynamic imaging studies and sonographic imaging are in the process of being perfected.

Thermography

Military technology has provided us with the knowledge to construct sophisticated infrared cameras, which can take images of the breast without the need for radiation exposure (X-rays) or breast tissue compression. These thermographic images are able to detect the heat signature of the increased blood flow associated with precancerous or malignant lesions.

In 1982, the Food and Drug Administration approved thermography as an adjunctive diagnostic breast screening procedure. The role of thermography has been misunderstood by many who compare its finding to that of the mammogram. This is like trying to compare apples to oranges. Breast thermography is a major risk indicator in that it can detect the first signs of cancerous processes long before a mass is noted on a mammogram. An abnormal thermogram indicates a ten times more significant risk for future breast cancer than a family history involving a mother or sister. Persistent abnormalities convey a twenty-two times higher risk for future breast cancer development.

Case Study: Importance of the Breast Surveillance Triad

To Kerri, age 57, breast health had become a major concern since her sister's breast cancer diagnosis two years ago, even though her own mammograms had always been normal. Last year she thought she had felt a thickening or lump in her right breast behind the nipple, but again her mammogram was normal and nothing further was suggested.

As part of her initial evaluation, a breast thermogram was performed. Normally, the temperature of both breasts, especially around the area of the nipples, should not differ by more than one degree Celsius. In Kerri's case the nipple of her right breast was more than two degrees Celsius warmer than the left.

The lymph nodes that drain the breast are located in the area under the arms known as the axilla. The axilla on her right side showed a warmer than expected signature, especially when compared with the left side. The thermogram indicated her risk for an abnormality was high for the right breast.

Kerri had already scheduled her yearly mammogram for that week and decided to keep the appointment. Even though the mammogram was read as normal, a sonogram of the right breast was taken because of the abnormal thermogram and the persistent palpable area. The sonogram showed "an irregular taller-than-wide solid mass, with angular and poorly defined margins measuring 10-20 millimeters that is seen in the right breast at three o'clock." A needle biopsy of this area at the time of the sonogram was positive for carcinoma. The increased infrared signature in the right axilla mentioned on the thermogram was later confirmed to be lymphatic spread of the breast cancer.

Kerri's case illustrates that there is no one perfect screening procedure. One must rely on the breast surveillance triad: a self-exam, an exam by a health practitioner, and a combination thermogram/mammogram screening.

The value of thermography is found in its ability to demonstrate the physiologic changes within the breast, while mammography demonstrates mostly anatomic changes. Physiologic changes can precede a detectable tumor (on mammogram or palpation) by seven to ten years. Early detection of these abnormal changes allows for the implementation of aggressive measures as described in this book, which are designed to reverse pre-cancerous processes. Remember, by the time a mass or a suspicious irregularity appears on a mammogram, one must proceed to intervention, which may involve surgery, chemotherapy, and/or radiation. It is much easier to prevent than to treat.

Thermography operates according to the following theory: Both pre-cancerous changes as well as cancers of the breast must have an increase in blood flow (compared with the normal surrounding tissue) in order to provide nutrients for rapid cell growth. The warmth of the blood appears in the form of infrared radiation that is emitted through the skin; therefore, the greater the flow of blood, the more infrared radiation will be irradiated from the overlying skin surface compared with the adjoining skin. Incredible as it may seem, the skin surface of the breast provides a looking glass as to what physiologic processes are occurring in the deeper tissue layers.

In addition, a thermogram allows the comparison of the infrared activity of one breast to the other.

Screening Mammograms

Traditional medicine currently favors the use of the mammogram as the primary tool for screening. As with estrogen replacement therapy, the news media has selectively disseminated information that has generated controversy and alarm as to the timing and reliability of mammograms.

Certainly, screening mammograms are not perfect. They can miss cancers, but it has been our experience that mammograms are capable of early detection of tumors that subsequently respond well to treatment. Most importantly, studies involving large groups of women point to the fact that mammogram screening can reduce the death rate from breast cancer by as much as 30 percent for women over age 50.

Mammograms/Thermograms:
The Warning Signs and Early Detection of Breast Cancer

Case Studies: Detection Is Good Protection

Rachel, 43 years old, had been seeing my associate for several years without any problems. She had declined to participate in our breast care program. Her initial mammogram was normal. Following this year's annual exam, a mammogram was ordered and revealed a "suspicious 9 millimeter mass in the 11 o'clock axis of the right breast, 3 centimeters from the nipple." The ultrasound-guided core biopsy of the mass was read by pathology as "infiltrating ductal carcinoma Grade 1." A lumpectomy was performed and no evidence was found of spread to the lymph nodes.

Beth, 54, had faithfully kept her annual mammogram appointments for the past seven years. Her latest mammogram, like all the others, was normal. Recently she had a breast exam as part of a pre-operative evaluation for cosmetic surgery. The physician had located a mass in the right breast, which was estimated to be 3 centimeters in size. The biopsy revealed "infiltrating lobular cancer," and she underwent bilateral radical mastectomies. Three lymph nodes were found to contain tumor cells on the affected side.

These cases reveal the diagnostic value as well as the potential shortcomings of mammograms. Better screening methods are needed and being developed. But in the meantime, the breast surveillance triad is the best overall approach.

Mammograms are X-rays that easily penetrate the transparent fat cells in the breast, but not denser objects such as calcium deposits, alveoli, ductal formations, and cystic or solid tumors. Premenopausal women tend to produce abundant amounts of estrogen and progesterone that convert large portions of the breast into the mammographically denser-appearing alveoli and ducts. The decrease in hormonal stimulation seen in postmenopause leads to a regression of these structures, with a simultaneous increase in less-dense fat cells.

Hormone replacement, especially with oral synthetic estrogens, can increase breast density, and mammogram studies have confirmed that a significant increase in density is a breast cancer risk factor. Therefore, mammograms can be used not only for detection of breast masses, but also conditions such as increases in breast density secondary to estrogen excess. This permits the implementation of our breast program to counter the unwanted overstimulation of breast tissues.

Many women may be concerned about the risks of X-ray radiation from mammograms. Let me put the risks into perspective. Modern mammograms expose you to relatively low levels of radiation — approximately 0.1 rads per image. This dose is equivalent to three months of everyday environmental background radiation or the same amount you could receive on a flight from New York to Los Angeles in a commercial airliner. The probability of this causing breast cancer is less than 1 in 25,000.

The consensus of the medical community is that the benefits of appropriately timed mammograms seem to far outweigh the risks. Consider this fact — that having a single mammogram every year from age 40 to age 90 exposes you to 0.01 percent of the radiation you would experience during treatment for breast cancer.

I, too, am concerned about damage to the breast cell and its matrix caused by simultaneous compression and exposure to mammographic-induced low-level radiation. The Committee on Biological Effects of Ionizing Radiation has stated, "There is no threshold below which exposure can be viewed as harmless." To minimize this radiation exposure, I suggest that individualized scheduling of mammograms be based on the breast surveillance program. Although a review of current studies concluded that mammogram radiation does not present a significant risk, the FEM Centre Breast Care Program is designed to reduce the potential tissue damage due to mammograms, high power lines, electric blankets, or any number of radiation sources existing in our high-tech society.

Self-Exam, Thermogram, Mammogram — Who and How Often?

Breast Self-Exam

At the age of twenty, a woman should begin a routine breast self-exam once a month.

Some investigators report that up to 56 percent of breast cancers are discovered by self-examination. For those women who still have menstrual cycles, the optimum window for breast exams is at the end of the menstrual flow.

Traditional medicine still views the mammogram as the gold standard in breast cancer detection. However, in order to avoid abnormal mammogram findings, one must rely on prevention, which requires the implementation of serial thermograms.

Thermograms

I suggest that a thermogram evaluation be obtained initially by women in their mid-thirties. This can be accomplished even earlier for those with breast pain or cystic changes. Serial follow-up is extremely helpful in ensuring resolution of inflammatory conditions.

Women 40 years and older should have yearly thermograms.

This provides us with the opportunity to detect those potential precancerous changes, which could progress to overt breast cancer over the next seven to ten years. The program described in this book can act as the primary intervention in the prevention of precancerous progression.

Mammograms/Thermograms:
The Warning Signs and Early Detection of Breast Cancer

Mammograms

Women age forty to forty-nine years should have screening mammograms every one to two years. (Recommended by the American College of Obstetricians and Gynecologists.)

There is some controversy over the routine screening of women ages forty to forty-nine. The Canadian National Breast Screening Study No. 1 found no reduction in breast cancer mortality by performing mammograms in this age group, but critics have cited flaws in the Canadian study that render its conclusion doubtable. Therefore, in the absence of periodic thermography, consideration should be given to the American College of Obstetricians and Gynecologists' recommendation for screening every one to two years in women of this age.

Women fifty and older should have an annual mammogram. (Currently, no consensus exists as to what age these exams can be stopped.)

In our clinical experience at the FEM Centre, we've documented that mammogram screenings of women in their forties (who were not on our Breast Care Program and had not obtained a thermogram) have resulted in the discovery of early breast cancers that were too small to be detected by clinical exam. In the absence of thermography, my concern is that waiting to begin screening mammograms until patients were age fifty could have allowed these cancers to grow for seven or eight years.

It is reasonable to start mammogram screening in the forty- to forty-nine-year range. Screening below the age of forty should be based on a family history of breast cancer. The usual recommendation is to begin mammogram screening five years before the age at which the youngest, premenopausal, first-degree relative was diagnosed with breast cancer.

Mammograms/Thermograms:
The Warning Signs and Early Detection of Breast Cancer

To decrease the incidence of breast cancer, I suggest the frequent use of thermograms to detect pre-cancerous changes and, if present, monitor their resolution using the FEM Centre Breast Care Program. Suspicious lesions detected by thermography require appropriate follow-up. An individualized program regarding the use of mammograms is important in order to detect anatomic lesions, which could require further intervention. Frequent breast self-exams comprise the third part of our multimodal approach.

Almost 95 percent of early stage breast cancers can be detected using our breast surveillance program. Just as important, however, is the potential to recognize and treat precancerous lesions years before they turn into cancer.

CHAPTER 12

Male Wellness: Being a Partner in Health

Because of a heightened public awareness of breast cancer, wellness and disease prevention have become especially important to women. However, in men as well as women, heart disease, depression, arthritis, diabetes, cancer, and even osteoporosis (nearly one-third of all osteoporotic fractures occur in men) are at epidemic levels. Prostate cancer is increasing at three times the rate of breast cancer, with both having similar causes — estrogen imbalances and toxicity.

After providing health care for enlightened women for more than twenty-five years, I have come to realize that the identical preventive concepts discussed in this book can be extended to their husbands or male companions, too.

Many times I have been asked, "Now, I feel great, but I'm worried about my husband. What can we do for him?"

Traditional medicine has placed comparatively little emphasis on male wellness and disease prevention. Men face essentially the same issues as women, but men tend to die sooner and live sicker. In fact, the United States ranks fifteenth in the world in terms of male longevity.

Social mores dictate that men avoid the doctor until faced with severe enough symptoms to prevent them from going to work. Most men are afraid they will be labeled as "chronic complainers" (an affront to one's masculinity) and instead will try to work through the pain. To men the terms "prevention" and "male hormonal balancing" can be quite alien, but they are just as important for men as they are for women. While it is acceptable to address chest pain, few midlife males will seek medical advice about issues such as:

- Lack of endurance/fatigue

- Problems maintaining an erection/a decrease in spontaneous morning erections

- Increasing weight gain

- Fuzzy memory

- Decreased urinary stream/frequent urination at night

- Depression

- Overcoming the, "Is this all that there is to look forward to for the rest of my life?" syndrome that in many cases leads to marital problems

- Insomnia

- Muscle aches

Approximately 30 million men in the United States (57 million by 2020) are between the ages of 45 and 55. During this time interval, men can go through a hormonal transition that is in many ways similar to that of a woman entering menopause. If your husband has at least three of the nine symptoms above, then he probably has already entered this hormonal transition.

These symptoms are warning signs of functional problems that, if not properly addressed, can result in the chronic diseases of aging. It is the decline in testosterone, in particular, that leads to the hormonal imbalances in what is termed *viropause, andropause,* or *male menopause.*

Whereas the precipitous decline in estrogen signals the onset of a woman's menopausal symptoms, the decline in a man's testosterone is associated with andropause and occurs gradually over a period of ten to fifteen years. During this time, a man's testosterone level may decline by up to 50 percent or more. That can lead to an increased risk for heart disease, depression, and even prostate cancer.

Significant health risks have been associated with andropause: a greater risk for heart disease independent of cholesterol and blood pressure; a greater risk for prostate cancer; and a higher incidence of depression, just to name a few.

Other hormones such as thyroid hormone, DHEA, pregnenolone, melatonin, and human growth hormone also decline in men. Many women who are left wondering, "What happened to the man that I married?" need to understand the personality and physical changes that result from andropause. As in menopause, andropause symptoms originate from both hormonal imbalances and a need for detoxification.

Hormonal balancing in men involves the use of bio-identical hormones such as testosterone that are usually applied as a gel to the skin daily or by injections. The testosterone level should be monitored through blood testing to arrive at an optimal and safe concentration. Restoring testosterone can dramatically improve a man's moods, energy levels, athletic ability, mental acuity, and sexual desire and performance.

While estrogen levels decline in women beginning with their menopausal transition, estrogen levels tend to rise in midlife men. Elevated estrogen can lead to breast development in men (gynecomastia) with an associated increase in the possibility of breast cancer, an increase in the risk of heart disease, an enlargement of the prostate (benign prostatic hypertrophy), and even an increased incidence of prostate cancer. (In terms of cancer causes, the prostate gland responds adversely to many of the same substances as the breast.)

Although seldom discussed, men can also develop breast cancer. For every one hundred women in the United States who are diagnosed with breast cancer, one male will develop the equivalent disease. As with women, the rate of male breast cancer is also increasing. Risk factors include: an imbalance of hormones such as estrogen, genetics, age (the average of onset is 65 years), ethnicity, and a toxic environment. Presentation of a hard, irregular, non-painful mass underneath the nipple should be regarded as suspicious. Men should routinely examine their breast for masses (and testicles to rule out testicular cancer). Following the suggestions discussed in this book provides an excellent means of prevention. Detection and treatment methods are similar to those used for female breast cancer.

The same hormones we evaluated in women in Chapter 9 — estradiol, thyroid hormones, DHEA, pregnenolone, melatonin, and human growth hormone — should also be evaluated in men. Treatment (excluding estrogen and progesterone) also is remarkably similar.

Exercise, stress reduction, and nutrition form the base of the wellness pyramid for men as well as women. In order to provide protection for the prostate, supplements are also important and should include omega-3 fatty acids (fish oil), multivitamins, plus those needed for regulating estrogen and promoting the health of the intestines (i.e., BreastSecure and IntestRestore). Resveratrol, which is found in red wine extract, has been cited as particularly helpful in protecting prostatic tissue. *Note: See Appendix E for a source for BreastSecure, IntestRestore, high-quality fish oil, and multivitamins.*

As men age, prostate enlargement can result in a weak urinary stream with frequent urination. DIMN, calcium D-glucarate, and red wine extract not only act to relieve this condition but also protect prostate cells from turning cancerous as a result of excessive estrogen. We have also noticed an improvement in the age-related increase in prostate size (benign prostatic hypertrophy) using our wellness program. Additionally, DIMN and calcium D-glucarate act on the cellular level to protect the prostate, heart, and brain.

I also suggest that daily supplementation include:

- Saw palmetto — 320 mg

- Lycopene — 10 to 15 mg; frequent use of tomato paste is even better

- Zinc — 40 to 50 mg

- Selenium — 200 to 400 mcg

- Vitamin E — 200 to 400 iu (in a mixture of both alpha and gamma forms)

Traditional medicine recommends that men who reach the age of fifty have a regular prostate exam along with a screening colonoscopy and a blood test for PSA, prostate-specific antigen. I would follow this with the FEM Centre's wellness regime of detoxification and chelation, again because we want to emphasize prevention over intervention after the fact.

Men tend to develop more plaque deposits in the arteries of their heart, leading to cardiovascular disease — the No. 2 killer of men behind cancer. The fast, electron-beam computed tomography unit (EBCT) is now available to scan the heart and detect calcium deposits in the coronary arteries long before symptoms develop. However, the most effective way to avoid heart disease is to remove the precursors.

The best place to start is our 21-day detoxification program, using medical food powders such as IntestRestore in conjunction with long-term chelation therapy. In addition, cardiologists have shown that using a lecithin-based liposomal EDTA supplement can help control cholesterol, diabetes, blood flow to the heart muscle, and high blood pressure.

The final reason (and most important one) men should consider this wellness program — your female partner!

It stands to reason that any of us, man or woman, has a diminished chance of success in a wellness program if our partner is out of balance hormonally and suffers from the same toxicities. So for men, sharing in her quest for a healthier mind and body by following the same program will not only provide her with the support she needs, but you will also enjoy the same benefits of a longer, healthier, and happier life.

Case Study: Partners in Health

Stephanie, at age 50, began to notice her menstrual flows were further apart, sometimes being absent for two months at a time. She began having night sweats, and suffering fatigue and mood swings. Her weight steadily climbed until now it was approaching 200 pounds. Neither exercise nor dieting seemed to help, which only added to her frustration.

Her husband, Rick, accompanied her to the FEM Centre, where a hormonal assessment revealed that Stephanie was entering late perimenopause. Also, her estrogen, DHEA, testosterone, and thyroid blood levels were insufficient. Stephanie scored a 25 on her detox questionnaire, indicating severe toxicity. This contributed to both weight gain and lack of energy. With this information in hand, she began our detox and hormone balancing programs.

Although somewhat hesitant, Rick went along with the new detoxification diet because Stephanie not only wanted to improve her own health, she also wanted Rick to stay fit. Plus, preparing the same foods for both, rather than a healthy meal for Stephanie and a standard American diet for her husband, would be easier. They also agreed to begin an exercise regimen.

After six weeks, Stephanie's labs showed dramatic improvement, and at fourteen weeks she had lost 12 pounds and Rick had lost 10. With this success, Rick began thinking about his state-of-health. For the past few years he had noticed a decrease in his activity level, a feeling of "burnout" with his job, general anxiety, and difficulty maintaining an erection. Stephanie and Rick decided he should have his hormones checked.

Rick's initial testosterone level was 251 g/dL (the normal level being 241 to 827 ng/dL) and a DHEA of 71 mg/dL (normally 70 to 310 mg/dL). While technically in the normal range, men with testosterone levels in the lower quartile do not function as well as those in the mid- to upper-normal ranges. Rick was placed on bio-identical testosterone and a DHEA supplement as part of our program designed for men. Six weeks later, his labs showed a testosterone level of 521 ng/dL and a DHEA of 222 mg/dL. When questioned at this visit he responded, "Everything seems to be working much better."

Rick and Stephanie have continued the wellness program for over six months resulting in additional weight loss and improved health for each. Rick's participation reinforces Stephanie's, and vice versa, creating a true win-win solution — partners in health.

CHAPTER 13

Breast Cancer Survivors

The purpose of this book is to reduce the chances of succumbing to breast cancer, but for the breast cancer survivor, the goal is to reduce your chances for recurrence.

Thanks to recent advances in medical science, the number of breast cancer survivors is increasing. We are getting better at treating breast cancer. However, for those who have had successful treatment or those who are concerned about getting cancer, a lifestyle change is mandatory.

Case Study: Avoiding Recurrence

Martha, now 56 years of age, was diagnosed with breast cancer around ten years ago. Having responded successfully to standard medical treatments, she was followed by an oncologist for the next five years without apparent recurrence of the cancer.

Four months before she came to the FEM Centre, she went to her family doctor with a case of bronchitis. When antibiotics failed to resolve the bronchitis, her physician ordered a chest X-ray, which revealed multiple pulmonary masses. Further examination showed the cancer had returned and now infiltrated not only her lungs but her liver as well.

How often have we heard this tragic story of someone who apparently had been free of breast cancer for five or ten years only to suffer a recurrence in the bone, lung, liver, brain, or other region of the body? The question is: How could this have been prevented?

When she arrived at the FEM Centre I reviewed her medical history. It showed Martha had received excellent care and responded to her cancer treatments with apparent remission of the tumor. Her follow-up visits to the oncologist were scheduled at yearly intervals and directed primarily toward cancer surveillance. When I asked Martha what preventive measures had been discussed following treatment, she looked at me quizzically and said, "Nothing was ever mentioned."

This highlights what I think is one of the principal weaknesses in the traditional approach to managing cancer. While the initial treatments are quite effective at killing tumor cells, there is far too little guidance offered on what should be done to prevent recurrences.

Initially, it is quite common for the original tumor to shower the body with microscopic clumps of cancer cells. *Metastasis* is the term used to describe this malignant characteristic. Those tissues containing the greatest amount of blood flow generally have the highest chance of being infiltrated. Traditional medicine attempts to kill these metastatic cancer cells using combinations of surgery, radiation, immunotherapy, and chemotherapy. Yet, even using the most resourceful treatments available, it is impossible to eradicate every cancer cell.

Traditional medicine views cancer only as disease of the individual cell caused by mutated or damaged DNA. This offers a partial explanation of the problem but leaves many issues unresolved, as we see in Martha's case. To prevent those metastatic cancer cells still present after traditional medical treatment from growing into tumors, we need to understand the function of the cellular matrix (as described in Chapters 2 and 8 and in the works of Drs. Sonnenschein and Pischinger listed in the bibliography).

The matrix, which envelops all normal cells, not only houses components of the immune system but also acts as a restraint for preventing excessive cell division. Every cell in the body must be restrained to some degree because each carries the basic genetic command to divide and evolve. According to cellular matrix theory, cancer cells arise from the breakdown of this harnessing mechanism, allowing uncontrolled growth.

A healthy matrix is able to restrain a metastatic cancer cell, preventing its further growth into a tumor. Therefore, breast cancer cells that have lodged in a healthy matrix of another organ (lung, liver, brain, etc.) can coexist in a dormant state, side-by-side with normal cells, without health risks.

Problems can begin to occur with a breakdown in this protective envelope. Aging and repeated toxic insults (listed in previous chapters) can lead to the deterioration of the matrix over a period of years, permitting the cancer cells to break free from their biologic harness.

At the FEM Centre, we have cared for breast cancer survivors who have had small metastatic lesions, as shown on X-rays, in areas such as the spine that remained dormant for years. I believe that vigilance and careful adherence to proper nutrition, a healthy lifestyle, and regular exercise in conjunction with ongoing detoxification have been fundamental in reinforcing this dormancy because these actions help restore and maintain a healthy cell matrix.

I believe that a reconsideration of what leads to initial breast cancer formation can help prevent long-term recurrences. The key is not viewing cancer cells as isolated entities but understanding their interaction with the environment in which they exist. Therefore, rather than take a "wait-and-see" approach after treatment, I advocate that an aggressive nutrition- and detoxification-based prevention program be instituted.

Regenerating and maintaining the integrity of the cell matrix requires ongoing restoration of the liver intestinal detox system; chelation of heavy metals; and deep tissue cleansing as listed in Chapter 8. Infrared saunas, colon cleansing, traditional Chinese medicine including "cupping," and lymphatic drainage are important forms of mechanical cleansing. Homeopathic remedies arrived at by special biofeedback testing are also invaluable. Periodic use of intravenous high-dose vitamin C and minerals should be considered.

Breast cancer is a chronic disease, which must be kept in check, just as heart disease or diabetes. When one is diagnosed with diabetes or heart disease, major modifications in diet and lifestyle ensue to prevent further progression. Likewise, I believe drastic changes should take place when the diagnosis is cancer. Failure to make these changes could result in an uphill battle similar to what Martha now faces.

Breast cancer survivors, like all of us, must deal with the normal aging process, but in addition they must face the threat of recurrence. Whereas the majority of women diagnosed are already post-menopausal, a growing number are premenopausal, and as a result of chemotherapy, have suffered ovarian failure leading to menopausal symptoms. Quality of life becomes an important consideration, because those who were the youngest (premenopausal) tend to be the most debilitated by the sudden loss of estrogen.

The concept that estrogen replacement is strictly forbidden if one has had breast cancer has come under intense scrutiny. A growing body of evidence in the medical literature suggests that estrogen replacement therapy in a treated and apparently cancer-free woman does not seem to increase her chances of recurrence. Along these lines I point out the following circumstances in which increased estrogen does not appear to raise the risk of subsequent cancers:

- The survival for pregnant women with breast cancer is the same as non-pregnant women when corrected for stage and age.

- Pregnancies after breast cancer do not necessarily increase the recurrence rate.

- The presence of functional ovaries does not increase the recurrence rate.

Still, the breast cancer survivor can no longer be complacent, but must aggressively seek a healthier lifestyle.

Having breast cancer underscores imbalances within the body that have been present long before the cancer cell turned into a tumor. It takes a breast cancer cell seven to ten years to divide to the point that it is clinically detectable, which means that the actual causes have been present even longer.

After undergoing traditional medical therapy to destroy the breast cancer cells, it is important to undertake a breast care program. Breast cancer survivors should adhere to the FEM Centre Breast Care Pyramid (see Chapter 6) to facilitate conventional treatment and ensure permanent remission. The degree of compliance must be dramatic and continuous. It is my firm belief that a determined change in lifestyle, such as following the FEM Centre Breast Care Program, can markedly increase your margin of safety.

As of now, there is no cure for breast cancer, so one must change the processes within the body that gave rise to the initial malignancy. A change in diet, exercise, and emotional habits, along with instigating detoxification and appropriate nutritional supplements, is the best way to reduce the chances of a recurrence.

The FEM Centre Breast Care Program is designed to optimize the immune system and other important components of good health. Your first and best defense against breast cancer is your own immune system. It must be kept vigilant at all times.

The following items are important activities for every breast cancer survivor:

- **A healthy diet** is a must. (See Appendix B — the 21-Day Detoxification Diet.) Food is the most important and effective natural medicine. Avoid sugar, since cancer cells use sugar as a primary energy source. The Women's Intervention Nutrition Study found that a diet similar to the one described in this book cut the recurrence of breast cancer by 24 percent.

- **Weight control** is mandatory for the same reasons mentioned in conjunction with breast cancer prevention. Regulation of both insulin and estrogen levels is influenced primarily by your weight. The estrogens produced by your own fat cells are far more dangerous than those used in a well-designed hormonal replacement program. Fat cells also generate inflammatory hormones that stress the immune system and destroy the cellular matrix (the tissue that surrounds the cell).

- **Exercise and stress reduction** are not an option, but a necessity. Exercise improves every aspect of your health, whereas stress has debilitating effects, both physically and mentally. Thankfully, a good exercise program has been shown to reduce stress.

- **Detoxification** is the key to cleaning out your body and balancing your immune system. The goal of detoxification is to lower the amount of toxins that have accumulated within the cellular matrix, allowing cells to communicate with their neighbors.

Health begins in the colon, which requires the use of our C.A.N. Program (Cleanse-Add-Nourish) frequently. I also suggest the daily use of IntestRestore (see Appendix C). Cleansing may need to be more rigorous for breast cancer survivors, in order to reverse the cancer-causing chronic imbalances, and should be supervised by a knowledgeable health care practitioner.

This program recommends that every woman assess (and if excessive, decrease) the heavy metal load in her body, and breast cancer survivors should give top priority to chelation therapy.

- **Hormonal balancing** is beneficial for breast cancer survivors, but the role of estrogen must be approached differently. Experimental studies have raised the concern that hormones such as pregnenolone, DHEA, and testosterone can be metabolized into estradiol, thus stimulating latent breast cancer cells to grow. On the other hand, we have found no increase in estradiol blood levels of breast cancer survivors after using low-dose bioidentical preparations of these hormones. As mentioned previously, DHEA and testosterone actually inhibit the growth of breast cancer cells. Should one still be concerned, an alternative is a low-dose methyltestosterone and/or 7-keto DHEA, neither of which can convert to estradiol. (Unfortunately, levels of these two hormone substitutes cannot be measured in standard laboratories.)

- **Thermography** should be performed with increasing frequency if breast tissue is present. Changes in blood flow patterns in the remaining tissue alert one to the need for more aggressive preventive measures and further evaluation.

Symptoms that become incapacitating, such as combinations of night sweats, daytime hot flashes, insomnia, bladder problems, memory issues, depression, and vaginal dryness (painful intercourse), may lead one to consider the use of estrogen replacement. While breast cancer recurrence is a main concern, the breast cancer survivor must also consider the preventive properties of estrogen replacement as it relates to heart disease, dementia, Alzheimer's, osteoporosis, and bladder urgency.

The most common forms of bio-identical estrogens we use are estriol-only or triest/biest preparations. Such preparations are generally weighted more in favor of estriol than estrone/estradiol.

The criteria for the use of low-dose, bio-identical estrogen replacement is:

- Non-hormonal treatment has failed to improve the quality of life.

  We have had great success with Chinese herbal medicine in the treatment of hot flashes and night sweats. The following herbs address the root of the problem by moistening and nourishing body fluids such as the blood (this is termed Yin fluids).

  – Di Gu Pi- cortex of wolfberry root

  – Bai Shao- white peony root

  – Sheng Di- Chinese foxglove root

  – Fu Xiao Mai- light wheat grain

  These herbs are generally not used alone but are combined into various formulations.

  Unlike black cohosh and red clover, there are no estrogen effects upon the breast cells.

- The patient must be determined to be cancer-free by her oncologist and have a low risk of recurrence.

- The patient fully understands the potential risks (as listed by the FDA) of taking estrogen.

  Absolute contraindications to estrogen replacement

  – unexplained vaginal bleeding

  – active liver disease

  – breast carcinoma

– active thrombophlebitis

– pregnancy

- The patient closely adheres to the FEM Centre Breast Care Program, especially the breast care nutrients (see Chapter 10) that are one of the keys to modulating estrogen's effect on breast tissue. This is of particular importance to the breast cancer survivor since it is the estrogen that your body makes that is most dangerous.

The goals are to:

- Increase the production of the 2-hydroxyestrogen that can kill breast cancer cells.

- Control the activity of the estrogen-producing enzyme aromatase to prevent the buildup of excess estrogen in the body.

- Ensure that breast cells maintain their ability to undergo apoptosis (programmed cell death).

- Protect the breast cell's DNA from damage and enable the cell to recognize and communicate with its neighboring cells.

- Decrease inflammation and cleanse the breast cell matrix by means of detoxification.

Additionally, it is important for your health practitioner to consider measuring your 2-hydroxy:16alpha-hydroxyestrogen ratio, obtain an iodine load test, and evaluate blood levels of vitamin D.

A combination of a healthy diet, weight control, exercise, stress reduction, detoxification, hormonal balancing, and the recommended breast care nutrients not only improves the health of your breasts, but greatly contributes to your overall health.

Being proactive in your health maintenance is a positive step, both physically and mentally. Our program provides all the necessary tools for a breast cancer survivor, allowing you to leave behind the victim mentality and become an active participant in your own recovery.

EPILOGUE

One day as I was driving to my office, in Fort Worth's downtown medical district, it dawned on me that the majority of new construction in the area had been of medical facilities treating only cancer or heart disease. Two of the hospitals near my office had just finished extensive construction projects devoted solely to cardiac patients, while local oncology groups were forced to expand and build new facilities thousands of square feet in size. A check with hospital districts in other cities revealed similar types of construction. Yes, these expansions were driven by a demand for services, which I find to be a sobering indicator of what lies in store for an aging population.

Other areas of the health care industry that have tapped into this thriving need for service include the pharmaceutical companies. New drugs are continually being introduced into the marketplace. Many of them are expensive and no more effective than the ones they are replacing. Plus, there seems to be a great deal of duplication (how many different synthetic hormonal preparations do we really need?)

In the highly competitive health care market, aggressive advertising campaigns on television and in magazines encourage people to ask their doctor whether a certain medication would be right for them. I was astonished one day while watching a television commercial that listed the benefits of a particular pain-relieving drug while showing a satisfied, pain-free patient. Toward the end of the commercial, the announcer stated, "This drug may cause liver or kidney failure and even death. Ask your doctor if this medication is appropriate for you."

Another recurring theme: Serious side effects being reported after a drug has been on the market for a number of years. As I tell my patients, you most likely will pay a price when relying only on pharmaceutical medications. Moreover, synthetic hormonal preparations and their adverse side effects are continually making headlines. (Upon opening the newspaper recently, I saw this headline in bold-faced letters: "Hormone pills on 'carcinogenic' list." Unfortunately, no distinction was made between synthetic pharmaceutical versus natural, or bio-identical, "hormone pills.")

I pose a simple question — how can a synthetic hormone that has taken an average of ten years to develop in a laboratory be better for your health and well-being than a hormone that nature has cultured over millions of years through evolution?"

Maybe it is time to regroup and reconsider our priorities. Using the wisdom of nature in the form of a bio-identical hormone replacement program, I have witnessed the fabulous results thousands of women have experienced not only in menopause and postmenopause but also in premenopause and younger. It is possible to turn back the biologic clock and once again experience vitality, clarity of thought, and a sense of well-being. Life does not have to revolve around a medicine cabinet.

Over a period of time we have noticed other benefits of our wellness program: Women were able to reduce or eliminate the pharmaceutical medications they were taking. For many patients, the initial visit may have been directed toward hormonal issues, but after following our program, chronic conditions such as fibromyalgia, gastrointestinal disorders such as irritable bowel syndrome, depression, diabetes, and arthritis seemed to improve dramatically.

The fear of breast cancer continues to overshadow the use of hormonal therapy. Yet, our blending of hormone replacement and detoxification into a wellness program has proved to be a powerful deterrent not only to breast cancer but to other cancers including ovarian. We also have observed a general decline in the numbers of other chronic diseases. Quite possibly the need for many of these new medical buildings and pharmaceutical drugs would decrease if more time and resources were directed toward investigating causes instead of chasing symptoms.

There will be new medical treatments offering solutions to many of the problems of aging that we currently confront. One of these that I find most interesting is in the emerging field of "regenerative medicine," which necessitates the use of stem cell therapy and genetic engineering. Although in its infancy, stem cell research is providing many intriguing insights into reversing the chronic disease process. Animal studies have suggested that stem cells can fix a broken brain or heart while providing unlimited possibilities for other body organs. Even now, amazing results have been reported in humans with advanced cancer.

Aging has been attributed to hormonal imbalances created either by glandular failure or the brain's insensitivity to hormone levels. Someday, stem cells may offer the ultimate way to balance hormones through the use of regenerative means to restore proper function to both aging endocrine glands and the brain's neurocircuits.

The future of regenerative medicine holds great potential for extending both our life and health span; however, we cannot abandon basic wellness tenets, as found in the adage, "let food be your medicine and let medicine be your food."

It is a blending of both the old and new ways that will strike a perfect balance for optimal health and wellness.

APPENDIX A

Detoxification Questionnaire
(Toxic Gut Survey—"Are you on fire?")

Digestion
- Heartburn
- Bloating
- Constipation
- Diarrhea
- Stomach cramps
- Excessive weight gain
- Food cravings
- Water retention/swelling
- Allergies/reactions to food
- Foul-smelling stools

Body Systems
- Joint aches/stiffness
- Headaches
- Rashes, hives
- Muscle aches
- Irregular heartbeat
- Chronic cough
- Weakness
- Frequent sore throats
- Itchy, swollen eyes
- Ringing in ears
- Ear and sinus infections
- Frequent vaginal yeast infections
- Excessive perspiration
- Acne
- Dark circles under eyes
- Persistent nail bed fungus

Emotions
- Mood swings
- Depression
- Irritable, jittery
- Anxious

Mental
- Poor concentration
- Fainting
- Numbness (hands/feet)
- Memory loss
- Poor hand-eye coordination

Medical Conditions
- Removal of gallbladder, or gallbladder disease
- Crohn's disease, lupus
- Psoriasis, eczema, rosacea
- Diverticular disease
- Irritable bowel syndrome

Circle each symptom or medical condition that currently applies to you. Your score is the total number of items you have circled. The following page provides an explanation of your score.

If your score is 9 or less, your toxicity levels appear to be mild to moderate. You should begin the *21-Day Detoxification Diet* (see Appendix B) to cleanse your entire system, and repeat this diet every three to six months. Otherwise, continue good eating habits and avoid those things discussed in Appendix C under "Plus Things to Avoid."

If your score totaled 10 or more, your toxicity levels are of greater concern. You should begin the *21-Day Detoxification Diet* and follow up with a health practitioner who is knowledgeable in cleansing. A formal chelation program should also be considered.

Note: on average, your body requires <u>one month of detoxification for every year</u> you have experienced the above symptoms.

APPENDIX B

The 21-Day Detoxification Diet

This diet is designed to eliminate many food-related gastrointestinal toxins that have accumulated within your body over the years. It is not to be confused with fad or other diets that have been popularized by the press.

Although a side effect of the detoxification plan is healthy weight loss, its primary purpose is cleansing. It is important to note that in cases where severe toxicity is indicated (see Appendix A — Detoxification Questionnaire), one should begin this diet slowly. It takes time to develop impaired metabolic function, and it requires time to heal.

After completion, one should repeat this program, at a minimum, several times yearly, and follow our long-term dietary suggestions in the interim.

Hypoallergenic naturopathic medicinal food powder

Start with the daily use of a hypoallergenic medical food powder that is specially formulated to restore and support the intestinal lining while reducing generalized inflammation. From the many brands to choose from we recommend IntestRestore. *Note: See Appendix E for a source for IntestRestore.*

Start slowly by mixing one to two scoops daily in cold water, or use the recipes provided below. Increase to two scoops twice daily after one week. IntestRestore may be taken alone or with meals.

Due to its continual intestinal support and anti-inflammatory properties, you should continue to use two scoops daily even after finishing the 21-day program.

Day 1 to Day 10

Note: "Real" food as opposed to processed food is distinguished by whether it can be picked, gathered, milked, fished, or hunted. Don't overeat. Chew thoroughly and thoughtfully. Rotate your food choices daily.

Avoid all grains, enriched and white flour, dairy products, legumes (beans), sweets, salt and foods containing salt, corn and corn products, soy, and animal proteins. Rice is the preferred protein source — it avoids soy-induced allergies.

Consume the following approved foods in the amounts stated:

- **Rice** — Hypoallergenic rice protein shake mix — 10 to 20 grams per serving, two servings daily. (This is also an ingredient in IntestRestore.)

- **Fruits** are complex carbohydrates in their whole form because they contain fiber, but they can be high in simple sugars. Eat only one or two servings (serving size: 1/2 cup) of fruits daily, but avoid the consumption of those with a high glycemic index. (See Appendix D — The Glycemic Index.)

- **Vegetables** — Non-starchy vegetables are an excellent source of natural fiber, vitamins, and minerals. It is recommended that you consume no less than five servings daily with at least two servings (serving size 1 cup) at lunch and at dinner. Recommendations for preparation include: raw, steamed, sautéed, roasted, used in soups, or as vegetable pâtés. Salads should be consumed daily. They are a quick and fresh source of dark leafy greens. *Note: Avoid starchy tubers such as potatoes, yams, and sweet potatoes.*

- **Nuts and seeds** are a great source of protein, but they are high in calories, so use in moderation, no more than one or two small, Dixie Cup portions daily. (One Dixie cup equals approximately 2 ounces.)

- **Oils** —Serving size: 1 to 2 tablespoons for cooking, dressings, and supplementation (no more than twice daily).

    – Avocado

    – Canola

    – Olive

    – Flaxseed

    – Walnut

Day 11 to Day 21

After ten days of the above foods only, add limited amounts of the animal proteins listed below:

- **Fish** — Serving size: 3 to 4 ounces; can be eaten up to two to three times weekly. Avoid those contaminated with mercury.

- **Meat** — Serving size: 3 ounces; three times per week or less; use leanest and cleanest (free range) available.

    – Beef (grass-fed sirloin and select "round" cuts)

    – Lamb shank, chops

    – Buffalo

    – Venison

    – Ostrich

    – Emu

- **Poultry** — Serving size: 3 to 4 ounces; three or four times per week

  – Chicken or turkey breast (free range; white meat only)

  – Game hen breast

- **Dairy/Eggs**

  – Free-range eggs, up to six per week

  – Full-fat kefir cheese, 2 to 3 ounces daily, or liquid kefir, up to ½ cup daily

  – Full fat yogurt (plain, organic)

  – Fresh organic butter and ghee, 1 tablespoon daily

- **Beverages**

  – Water (filtered), 64 to 128 ounces per day

  – Green tea (3 cups daily)

  – Cranberry juice (unsweetened)

  – Mineral water

  (Avoid alcohol)

Recipes that can be used starting on Day 11

Rockin' Raspberry Smoothie

1 to 2 scoops IntestRestore
4 ounces raspberries
¼ to ⅓ cup full-fat plain organic yogurt or kefir
½ cup ice
Water (filtered) added to desired consistency
1 tablespoon omega 3-6-9 oil

Strawberry Almond Super Protein Shake

1 to 2 scoops IntestRestore
½ to 1 cup fresh strawberries
¼ cup almonds (blend very well)
½ teaspoon vanilla
½ teaspoon cinnamon
1 scoop whey protein concentrate (about 20 grams) (optional)
1 tablespoon omega 3-6-9 oil
½ cup ice
Unsweetened soymilk for lighter consistency
Stevia to taste

Other additions:	*Other fruits for base:*
Rice bran	Peaches
Green food powder	Mangoes
Egg yolks or whites	Cranberries

Listed below are the supplements that are included in Intest-Restore, which by supporting the liver-intestinal detoxification system not only protects the breasts, but also the heart, brain, and bones.

Beta-sitosterol is a plant sterol that has anti-inflammatory, cancer-fighting, and immune-modulating effects. (It also improves prostatic function and has been shown to reduce elevated cholesterol levels.)

L-glutamine is the most abundant amino acid in the bloodstream and is used by intestinal cells (enetrocytes) as their primary source of fuel.

L-glycine is an amino acid that reduces gastric distress, improves detoxification in the liver, increases the release of human growth hormone, and balances the immune system.

Methylsulfonylmethane (MSM) is a primary source of bioavailable sulfur, which is usually removed by the industrial/commercial processing of food. MSM improves digestive tract problems and enhances the liver's ability to remove toxins from your body by sulfation. It also helps eradicate yeast overgrowth in the colon—especially after use of antibiotics.

N-acetyl-cysteine (NAC) increases the production of the powerful antioxidant glutathione, and shows potential as a preventive agent in cancers such as breast cancer.

Quercitin is widely distributed in the plant kingdom and provides many benefits including heart protection, cancer prevention, and antiviral and anti-inflammatory effects. Quercitin attaches to estrogen binding site 2, which inhibits overstimulation of the breast cell by estradiol.

Boswella has powerful anti-inflammatory effects, especially in the intestines.

Tumeric is the active ingredient derived from the herb curcuma longa. The active constituents, which include curcumin, have been shown to be powerful antioxidants, which can protect the liver, fight cancer, and be anti-inflammatory. Cancer researchers have noted its chemopreventive and therapeutic properties. Recent studies have confirmed that it helps stop the spread of breast cancer cells to other areas of the body.

Slippery elm has been used by Native Americans as a soothing herb that provides fast-acting relief for digestive and bowel problems. It provides a protective coating for the intestinal lining.

Green tea extract consists of a group of polyphenols of which epigallocatechin-3-gallate (EGCG) is best known for preventing and fighting breast cancer. EGCG also enhances the growth of good bacteria in the intestines.

Alpha lipoic acid elevates levels of the antioxidant glutathione, which can inactivate dangerous estrogen metabolites (4OH).

Grape seed extract is derived from the small seeds of the red grape and is a rich source of flavonoids. The antioxidants in these seeds are said to be even more powerful than vitamins C and E. Grape seed extract helps prevent heart disease and deters breast cancer formation by inhibiting aromatase.

Silymarin is the active constituent of milk thistle. It is a powerful protector and regenerator of the liver. Studies also suggest that it may inhibit a liver enzyme (CYP3A4) that produces estrogen metabolites dangerous to the breast.

Rosemary is a spice that has long been used in Ayurvedic medicine for anti-tumor effects. It is a potent anti-inflammatory herb that inhibits the COX-2 enzyme. Rosemary terpenes increase the production of the breast cancer-killing 2OH estrogen.

Ginger is a spice that contains powerful anti-inflammatory substances known as gingeroids. Inhibitors of COX-2 enzymes, gingeroids reduce inflammation and reduce the risk of cancer. Ginger prevents uncontrolled cell division by blocking tumor promoters such as epidermal growth factor.

Bromelain, which is a powerful enzyme derived from the pineapple plant, supports digestive health and lowers inflammation. Animal and human studies indicate its ability to prevent cancer metastasis.

Cinnamon is a culinary spice consisting of bioactive ingredients such as hydroxychalcone. These agents have a positive influence on insulin signaling to the cell and can reverse insulin resistance. Insulin insensitivity increases weight gain, especially around the midsection of the abdomen, disrupting hormonal balance and increasing the risk of breast cancer.

B vitamins — especially folic acid, B6, and B12 — are instrumental in the cancer-preventing methylation process. Elevated homocysteine levels, which have been linked to heart disease and even Alzheimer's, can be lowered using B vitamins. B5 (pantothenic acid) provides support for both the intestines and the adrenal glands.

APPENDIX C

Daily Regime and Regular Interval Regime (Plus Things to Avoid)

Daily

A long-term meal plan should include a predominantly plant-based, vegetarian diet: two-thirds vegetables plus one-third protein consisting of legumes, fish, turkey, chicken, soy, or lean red meat. *Avoid wheat and sweets.* For specific food choices I suggest you refer to the nutrition section of Chapter 7 or our 21-day Detoxification Diet in Appendix B.

Try to eat every three to four hours, which equals three meals a day with two snacks. Drink six to eight glasses of filtered water daily. Eat one bowl of slow cooked oatmeal twice weekly. Make a habit of taking one to two scoops of IntestRestore daily (mixed in water or blended in drinks such as smoothies) ideally, just before mealtime.

Practice the *Twenty-Minute Eating Rule*; it prevents you from eating too rapidly and subsequently consuming too much. Eat your meal over at least a twenty-minute period:

- Eat 25 percent of the meal in the first ten minutes

- Eat the next 25 percent over a five-minute period

- Eat the next 25 percent over a five-minute period

- If you're eating out, ignore the remaining 25 percent of the meal

- For a regular meal at home, finish eating the final 25 percent.

Begin Daily Healthy Habits:

Take good multivitamin (see Chapter 10) and/or IntestRestore along with the following Breast Care Nutrients:

- Omega-3 fish oil (1.5 to 3 grams of a combination of EPA and DHA)

- Iodine as determined by your health practitioner

- BreastSecure — which combines three nutritional, chemo-preventive supplements into an enhanced delivery system. Take one to two capsules daily with meals. BreastSecure includes:

    — DIMN

    — Red wine extract

    — Calcium D-glucarate

    Note: Appendix E lists sources for BreastSecure, IntestRestore, and high-quality fish oil.

Lifestyle Habits

- Exercise a total of 150 to 180 minutes per week.

- Aerobic exercise: Walk two and a half to three miles in thirty to forty-five minutes.

- Muscle exercise: resistance training (thirty to forty-five minutes) alone or combine with walking.

- Focus on stress reduction: "Happy thoughts make happy molecules." Take periodic breaks (five to twenty minutes each) daily out of your busy schedule to enjoy silence, deep breaths, and/or pleasant thoughts. Try to get five to ten minutes of sun exposure three times weekly. Be sure to allocate adequate amounts of *me* time.

- Do not eat two to three hours before bedtime.

Things to Avoid

- Sugar
- Carbohydrate-loaded cereals/enriched flour
- Fast and processed foods, and foods containing trans-fatty acids and/or hydrogenated oils (margarine)
- Excess ingestion of saturated fats
- Overcooked meat/microwaving, especially in plastic containers or covered with Saran Wrap
- Avoid food or water that has been frozen in plastic containers
- Smoking and secondhand smoke
- Excessive caffeine
- Alcohol
- Continuous use of underwire support bras
- Exposure to electromagnetic fields (high tension wires), petrochemicals, heavy metals, organochlorines (pesticides and dioxin), and air pollution
- Toxic thoughts

Regular Interval Regime for Breast Care

Breast Surveillance:

- Periodic thermograms/mammograms (see Chapter 11)

(American Cancer Society recommendations):

- Over age 20: Monthly breast self-exam (done just after finishing menstrual flow). Cancer generally presents as a solitary, painless, hard, non-movable mass. Only 10 percent of cancers are painful.

- Age 20 to 39: Every one to three years — a clinical breast exam by a health practitioner

- Age 40 and older: Once a year — a clinical breast exam

Hormonal Balance: Ongoing with the aid of a physician using bio-identical hormones.

Detoxification (Prevention)

Immediate — Things to Do Now!

Begin the 21-day detoxification program (see Appendix B) and repeat several times yearly. For treatment of chronic problems, you will need to follow a formal program that is supervised by a knowledgeable practitioner.

Long Term

Commit to a course of chelation. A convenient method is the use of an oral chelator such as a lecithin-based liposomal-encapsulated EDTA. For those preparations containing 1 to 2 grams of EDTA, use one vial weekly in divided doses for twenty-five to thirty weeks. This does not have to be done consecutively, but should be finished within twelve to eighteen months. Every three months thereafter, one vial should be used to prevent a re-accumulation of heavy metals. Intravenous chelation can also be used, especially for chronic conditions that include heart disease. Chelation programs should be managed only by trained practitioners. *Note: See Appendix E for a source for EDTA.*

APPENDIX D

The Glycemic Index

The higher the Glycemic Index number, the faster a food raises blood sugar. Conversely, the lower the Glycemic Index number, the slower blood sugar will rise. Obviously, the higher-number foods are to be avoided and the lower-number foods (rated 80 or less) are encouraged.

Vegetables and legumes (almost all vegetables have a very low Glycemic Index rating)

Artichoke (cooked) 25
Asparagus 22
Baked beans 70
Beets 68
Black-eyed peas 53
Broccoli (raw) 23
Brussels sprouts (raw) 23
Carrots 92
Cauliflower 21
Chickpeas (dried) 47
Corn 76
Garbanzo beans 64
Kidney beans (canned) 71
Lentils (green, dried) 36
Lima beans 46
Parsnips 96
Peas (green, dried) 50
Peas (frozen) 65
Pinto beans (canned) 64

Potato (instant mashed) 120
Potato (mashed) 117
Potato (new, white, boiled) 80
Potato (new, red, boiled) 70
Soy 20
Sweet potato 70
White beans (dried) 54
Yams 74

Cereals

All bran 74
Cornflakes 121
Muesli 96
Oat bran 85
Oatmeal (instant) 89
Oatmeal (slow-cooked) 49
Puffed rice 132
Puffed wheat 110
Shredded wheat 97

Cookies

Fat-free .... 100 +
Oatmeal 78
Shortbread 88
Water biscuits 100

Dairy

Custard 59
Ice cream 69
Ice cream (fat-free) .... 90 +
Milk (skim) 46
Milk (whole) 44

Yogurt (plain, full-fat) 52
Yogurt (with fruit, sugar) .... 90 +
Yogurt (frozen, fat-free) .... 90 +
Yogurt (with fruit, artificial sugar) 63

Fruits

Apple 49
Apple juice (unfiltered) 55
Applesauce 52
Apricot 73
Banana 82
Cherries 23
Dates 95
Grapefruit 26
Grapes 45

APPENDIX E

Resources

You can locate additional information and purchase BreastSecure and IntestRestore over the Internet at www.femcentre.com or call 1-888-FEMCNTR (1-888-336-2687).

High-quality fish oil, multivitamins, EDTA, and other supplements can be purchased over the Internet at www.femcentre.com.

You can find more information about thermography on the Internet at www.energyhealth.com.

Call FFP Laboratory at 1-877-900-5556 for more information about iodine-load testing.

More information about NeuroResearch and Dr. Marty Hinz's program can be found at www. neuroreplete.com.

BIBLIOGRAPHY

Abou-Issa H., Moeschberger M., et al. "Relative efficacy of glucarate on the initiation and promotion phases of rat mammary carcinogenesis." *Anticancer Research* 15(3) (1995): 805-10.

Abraham G.E., Flechas J.D., et al. "Orthoiodosupplementation: Iodine sufficiency of the whole human body." *Original Internist* 9(4) (2002): 30-41.

ACOG Practice Bulletin-Breast Cancer Screening. Number 42. April 2003.

Adlercreutz H., Pulkkinen. "Studies on the role of intestinal bacteria in metabolism of synthetic and natural steroid hormones." *Journal of Steroid Biochemistry* 20(1984): 217-219.

Alternative Medicine Review Monographs-Volume One. Alternative Medicine Review, 2002.

Ambrosone C.B., Freudenheim J.L., et al. "Cigarette smoking, N-acetyltransferase 2 genetic polymorphisms, and breast cancer risk." *Journal of the American Medical Association* 276(18) (1996): 1494-501.

Ardies C.M., Dees C. "Xenoestrogens significantly enhance risk for breast cancer during growth and adolescence." *Medical Hypotheses* 50(6) (1998): 457-64.

Ashfield-Watt P.A., Pullin C.H., et al. "Methylenetetrahydrofolate reductase 677C→T genotype modulates homocysteine responses to a folate-rich diet or a low dose folic acid supplement: a randomized controlled trial." *American Journal of Clinical Nutrition* 76(1) (2002): 180-6.

Awad A.B., Downie A.C., et al. "Inhibition of growth and stimulation of apoptosis by beta-sitosterol treatment of MDA-MB-231 human breast cancer cells in culture." *International Journal of Molecular Medicine* 5(5) (2000): 541-5.

Badawi A.F., Cavalieri E.L., et al. "Role of human cytochrome P450 1A1, 1A2, 1B1, and 3A4 in the 2-, 4-, and 16alpha-hydroxylation of 17beta-estradiol." *Metabolism* 50(9) (2001): 1001-3.

Bagchi D., Das D.K., et al. "Benefits of resveratrol in women's health." *Drugs in Experimental Clinical Research* 27(5/6) (2001): 233-248.

Bagis T., Gokcel A., et al. "The effects of short-term medroxyprogesterone acetate and micronized progesterone on glucose metabolism and lipid profiles in patients with polycystic ovary syndrome: a prospective randomized study." *Journal of Clinical Endocrinol Metabolism* 87(10) (2002): 4536-40.

Baker L., Meldrum K.K. "The role of estrogen in cardiovascular disease." *Journal of Surgical Research* 115(2) (2003): 325-44.

Barbosa-Silva M.C., Barros A.J., et al. "Bioelectrical impedance analysis in clinical practice: a new perspective on its use beyond body composition equations." *Current Opinion in Clinical Nutrition and Metabolic Care* 8(3) (2005): 311-7.

Barclay L. "Levonorgestrel IUDs may not adversely affect glucose metabolism in type 1 diabetes." *Current Opinion in Obstetrics and Gynecology* 105(2005): 811-15.

Behl C. "Estrogen can protect neurons: modes of action." *Journal of Steroid Biochemical Molecular Biology* 83(2002): 195-7.

Berges R.R., Windeler J., et al. "Randomized, placebo-controlled, double-blind clinical trial of beta-sitosterol in patients with benign prostatic hyperplasia." Beta-sitosterol Study Group. *Lancet* 345(8964) (1995): 1529-32.

Berstein L.M., Santen R.J. "Three-component model of oestrogen formation and regulation of intratumoural oestrogen pool in breast neoplasms." *Medical Hypotheses* 45(6) (1995): 588-90.

Berstein L.M., Tsyrlina E.V., et al. "Catecholestrogens excretion in smoking and non-smoking postmenopausal women receiving estrogen replacement therapy." *Journal of Steroid Biochemistry and Molecular Biology* 72(3) (2000): 143-7.

Bianco A.C., Salvatore D., et al. "Biochemistry, cellular and molecular biology, and physiological roles of the iodothyronine selenodeiodinases." *Endocrine Review* 23(1) (2002): 38-89.

Biancone L., Monteleone I. "Resident bacterial flora and immune system." *Digestive and Liver Disease* 34(Supplement 2) (2002): S37-43.

Bland, J., et al. *Clinical Nutrition: A Functional Approach.* The Institute For Functional Medicine, 1999.

Blumel J.E., Castelo-Branco C. "Effects of transdermal estrogens on endothelial function in postmenopausal women with coronary disease." *Climateric* 6(1) (2003): 38-44.

Blumer W., Cranton E.M. "Ninety percent reduction in cancer mortality after chelation therapy with EDTA." *Journal of Advancement in Medicine* 2 (1989): 183-8.

Bode A., Ma W., et al. "Inhibition of epidermal growth factor-induced cell transformation and activator protein 1 activation by [6]-Gingerol." *Cancer Research* 61(3) (2001): 850-3.

Borek C. "Dietary antioxidants and human cancer." *Integrative Cancer Therapies* 3(4) (2004): 333-41.

Bowes W.A., Katta L.R., et al. "Triphasic randomized clinical trial: Comparison of effects on carbohydrate metabolism." *American Journal of Obstetrics and Gynecology* 161(5) (1989): 1402-7.

Boyd N.F., Stone J., et al. "Dietary fat and breast cancer risk revisited: a meta-analysis of the published literature." *British Journal of Cancer* 89(9) (2003): 1672-85.

Bradley C.N., William J.K., et al. "Testosterone responses after resistance exercise in women: Influence of regional fat distribution." *International Journal of Sport Nutrition and Exercise Metabolism* 11(4) (2001): 451-65.

Bradlow H.L., Telang N.T., et al. "2-hydroxyestrogen: the 'good' estrogen." *Journal of Endocrinology* 150 Supplement (1996): S259-65.

Brinton R.D. "Impact of estrogen therapy on Alzheimer's disease: A fork in the road?" *CNS Drugs* 18(7) (2004): 405-422.

Brodie A.M., LU Q., Long B.J., et al. "Aromatase and COX-2 expression in human breast cancers." *Journal of Steroid Biochemistry and Molecular Biology* 79(1-5) (2001): 41-7.

Brooks J.D., Ward W.E., et al. "Supplementation with flaxseed alters estrogen metabolism in postmenopausal women to a greater extent than does supplementation with an equal amount of soy." *American Journal of Clinical Nutrition* 79(2) (2004): 318-25.

Browning L.M. "n-3 Polyunsaturated fatty acids, inflammation, and obesity related disease." *Proceedings of the Nutrition Society* 62(2) (2003): 447-53.

Brownstein, David. *Iodine: Why You Need It. Why You Can't Live Without It.* Medical Alternative Press, 2004.

Cal C., Garban H., et al. "Resveratrol and cancer: chemoprevention, apoptosis, and chemo-immunosensitizing activities." *Current Medicinal Chemistry. Anti-Cancer Agents* 3(2) (2003): 77-93.

Campbell I.G., Baxter S.W., et al. "Methylenetetrahydrofolate reductase polymorphism and susceptibility to breast cancer." *Breast Cancer Research* 4(6) (2002): R14.

Cann S., van Netten J.P., et al. "Hypothesis: Iodine, selenium and the development of breast cancer." *Cancer Causes and Control* 11(2) (2000): 121-127.

Casdorph, Richard, Morton Walker. *Toxic Metal Syndrome.* Avery, 1995.

Casson P.R., Andersen R.N., et al. "Oral dehydroepiandrosterone in physiologic doses modulates immune function in postmenopausal women." *American Journal of Obstetrics and Gynecology* 169(6) (1993): 1536-9.

Cavalieri E.L., Li K.M., et al. "Catechol orthoquinones: the electrophilic compounds that form depurinating DNA adducts and could initiate cancer and other diseases." *Carcinogenesis* 23(6) (2002): 1071-7.

Cavalieri E.L., Rogan E.G. "A unified mechanism in the initiation of cancer." *Annals of the New York Academy of Science* 959 (2002): 341-54.

Chang B.L., Zheng S.L., et al. "Polymorphisms in the CYP1B1 gene are associated with increased risk of prostate cancer." *British Journal of Cancer* 89(8) (2003): 1524-9.

Chang K.J., Lee T.Y., et al. "Influences of percutaneous administration of estradiol and progesterone on human breast epithelial cell cycle *in vivo.*" *Fertility and Sterility* 63(4) (1995): 785-91.

Chang Y.C., Riby J., et al. "Cytostatic and antiestrogenic effects of 2-(indol-3-ylmethyl)-3, 3'-diindolylmethane, a major *in vivo* product of dietary indole-3-carbinol." *Biochemical Pharmacology* 58(5) (1999): 825-34.

Chen D., Auborn K. "Fish oil constituent docosahexaenoic acid selectively inhibits growth of human papillomavirus immortalized keratinocytes." *Carcinogenesis* 20(2) (1999): 249-54.

Chen I., McDougal A., et al. "Aryl hydrocarbon receptor-mediated antiestrogenic and antitumorigenic activity of diindolylmethane." *Carcinogenesis* 19(9) (1998): 1631-9.

Chetrite G.S., Cortes-Prieto J., et al. "Comparison of estrogen concentrations, estrone sulfatase, and aromatase activities in normal, and in cancerous, human breast tissues." *Journal of Steroid Biochemistry and Molecular Biology* 72(1-2) (2000): 23-7.

Chlebowski R.T., Blackburn G.L., et al. "Dietary fat reduction improves relapse-free survival in postmenopausal women previously treated for early-stage breast cancer: Results from a phase III women's intervention nutrition study." *Clinical Breast Cancer* 6(2) (2005): 112-114.

Choe S.Y., Kim S.J., et al. "Evaluation of estrogenicity of major heavy metals." *Science of the Total Environment* 312(1-3) (2003): 15-21.

Clark L.C., Combs G.F Jr., et al. "Effects of selenium supplementation for cancer prevention in patients with carcinoma of the skin. A randomized controlled trial. Nutritional Prevention of Cancer Study Group." *Journal of the American Medical Association* 276(24) (1996): 1957-63.

Clarkson T.B. "Progestogens and cardiovascular disease. A critical review." *Journal of Reproductive Medicine* 44(2 Supplement) (1999): 180-4.

Clur A. "Di-iodothyronine as part of the oestradiol and catechol oestrogen receptor—the role of iodine, thyroid hormones and melatonin in the aetiology of breast cancer." *Medical Hypotheses* 27(4) (1988): 303-11.

Colditz G.A., Hankinson S.E., et al. "The use of estrogens and progestins and the risk of breast cancer in postmenopausal women." *New England Journal of Medicine* 332(24) (1995): 1589-93.

Cos S., Martinez-Campa C., et al. "Melatonin modulates aromatase activity in MCF-7 human breast cancer cells." *Journal of Pineal Research* 38(2) (2005): 136-42.

Coussens L.M., Werb Z. "Inflammation and Cancer." *Nature* 420(6917) (2002): 860-67.

Cranton, Elmer. *A Textbook on EDTA Chelation. 2nd edition.* Hampton Roads, 2001.

Csizmadi I., Collet J.P., et al. "The effects of transdermal and oral oestrogen replacement therapy on colorectal cancer risk in postmenopausal women." *British Journal of Cancer* 90(1) (2004): 76-81.

Cucinelli F., Soranna L., et al. "Estrogen treatment and body fat distribution are involved in corticotropin and cortisol response to corticotropin-releasing hormone in postmenopausal women." *Metabolism* 51(2) (2002): 137-43.

Cunningham, MacDonald, Gant, et al. *Williams Obstetrics. 20th edition.* Appleton and Lange, 1997.

Dawling S., Roodi N., et al. "Methoxyestrogens exert feedback inhibition on cytochrome P450 1A1 and 1B1." *Cancer Research* 63(12) (2003): 3127-32.

Decenzi A., Omodei U., et al. "Effect of transdermal estradiol and oral conjugated estrogen on C-reactive protein in retinoid-placebo trial in healthy women." *Circulation* 106(10) (2003): 127-8.

Derry, David. *Breast Cancer and Iodine.* Traaford, 2001.

Diamond, Jed. *Male Menopause.* Sourcebooks, 1998.

DiSaia P.J., Grosen E.A., et al. "Replacement therapy for breast cancer survivors. A pilot study." *Cancer* 76(10 Supplement) (1995): 2075-8.

Dubey R.K., Gillespie D.G., et al. "Methoxyestradiols mediate the antimitogenic effects of locally applied estradiol on cardiac fibroblast growth." *Hypertension* 39(2 Part 2) (2002): 412-7.

Bibliography

Dubey R.K., Gillespie D.G., et al. "CYP450-and COMT–derived estradiol metabolites inhibit activity of human coronary artery SMCs." *Hypertension* 41(3 Part 2) (2003): 807-13.

Dubey R.K., Tofovic S.P., et al. "Cardiovascular pharmacology of estradiol metabolites." *Journal of Pharmacology and Experimental Therapeutics* 308(2) (2003): 403-9.

Dunn J.F., Merriam G.R., et al. "Testosterone-estradiol binding globulin binds to 2-methoxyestradiol with greater affinity than to testosterone." *Journal of Clinical Endocrinology and Metabolism* 51(2) (1980): 404-6.

Eastman, A. "Cell cycle checkpoints and their impact on anticancer therapeutic strategies." *Journal of Cell Biochemistry* 91(2) (2004): 223-31.

Eden J., Wren B.G. "Hormone replacement therapy after breast cancer: a review." *Cancer Treatment Reviews* 22(5) (1996): 335-43.

Eng E.T., Williams D., et al. "Anti-aromatase chemicals in red wine." *Annals of the New York Academy of Science* 963 (2002): 239-46.

Eng E.T., Williams D., et al. "Suppression of aromatase (estrogen synthetase) by red wine phytochemicals." *Breast Cancer Research and Treatments* 67(2) (2001): 133-46.

Eng E.T., Ye J., et al. "Suppression of estrogen biosynthesis by procyanidin dimers in red wine and grape seeds." *Cancer Research* 63(23) (2003): 8516-22.

Epstein, Samuel, David Steinman, Suzanne Levert. *The Breast Cancer Prevention Program.* Macmillan USA, 1997.

Ernster V.L., Wrensch M.R., et al. "Benign and malignant breast disease: initial study results of serum and breast fluid analyses of endogenous estrogens." *Journal of the National Cancer Institute* 79(5) (1987): 949-60.

Escobar-Morreale H.F., del Rey F.E., et al. "Only the combined treatment with thyroxine and triiodothyronine ensures euthyroidism in all tissues of the thyroidectomized rat." *Endocrinology* 137(6) (1996): 2490-502.

Eskin B.A., Bartuska D.G., et al. "Mammary gland dysplasia in iodine deficiency. Studies in rats." *Journal of the American Medical Association* 200(8) (1967): 691-5.

Eskin B.A., Grotkowski C.E., et al. "Different tissue responses for iodine and iodide in rat thyroid and mammary glands." *Biological Trace Element Research* 49(1) (1995): 9-19.

Farzati A., Esposito K., et al. "Effects of transdermal hormone replacement therapy on levels of soluble P- and E-selectin in postmenopausal healthy women." *Fertility and Sterility* 77(3) (2002): 476-80.

Feigelson H.S., Coetzee G.A., et al. "A polymorphism in the CYP17 gene increases the risk of breast cancer." *Cancer Research* 57(6) (1997): 1063-5.

Fentiman I.S. "Timing of surgery for breast cancer." *International Journal of Clinical Practice* 56(3) (2002): 188-90.

Fineberg S.E. "Glycaemic control and hormone replacement therapy: implications of the Postmenopausal Estrogen/Progestogen Intervention (PEPI) study." *Drugs and Aging* 17(6) (2000): 453-61.

Fitzpatrick L.A., Pace C., et al. "Comparison of regimens containing oral micronized progesterone or medroxyprogesterone acetate on quality of life in postmenopausal women: a cross-sectional survey." *Journal of Women's Health and Gender-based Medicine* 9(4) (2000): 381-7.

Flake G.P., Andersen J., et al. Etiology and pathogenesis of uterine leiomyomas: a review." *Environmental Health Perspectives* 111(8) (2003): 1037-54.

Fleischauer A.T., Simonsen N., et al. "Antioxidant supplements and risk of breast cancer recurrence and breast cancer-related mortality among postmenopausal women." *Nutrition and Cancer* 46(1) (2003): 15-22.

Fohr I.P., Prinz-Langenohl R., et al. "5,10-methylenetetrahydrofolate reductase genotype determines the plasma homocysteine-lowering effect of supplementation with 5-methyltetrahydrofolate or folic acid in healthy young women." *American Journal of Clinical Nutrition* 75(2) (2002): 275-82.

Foidart J.M., Colin C., et al. "Estradiol and progesterone regulate the proliferation of human breast epithelial cells." *Fertility and Sterility* 69(5) (1998): 963-9.

Funahashi H., Imai T., et al. "Suppressive effect of iodine on DMBA-induced breast tumor growth in the rat." *Journal of Surgical Oncology* 61(3) (1996): 209-13.

Funahashi H., Imai T., et al. "Seaweed prevents breast cancer?" *Japanese Journal of Cancer Research* 92(5) (2001): 483-7.

Gago-Dominquez M., Yuan J.M., et al. "Opposing effects of dietary n-3 and n-6 fatty acids on mammary carcinogenesis: The Singapore Chinese Health Study." *British Journal of Cancer* 89(9) (2003): 1686-92.

Gambrell R.D. Jr., Maier R.C., et al. "Decreased incidence of breast cancer in postmenopausal estrogen-progestogen users." *Obstetrics and Gynecology* 62(4) (1983): 435-43.

Gao N., Nester R.A., et al. "4-hydroxyestradiol but not 2-hydroxy-estradiol induces expression of hypoxia-inducible factor 1alpha and vascular endothelial growth factor A through phosphatidylinositol 3-kinase/Akt/FRAP pathway in OVCAR-3 and A2780-CP70 human ovarian carcinoma cells." *Toxicology and Applied Pharmacology* 196(1) (2004): 124-35.

Gautherie M., Gros C.M. "Breast thermography and cancer risk prediction." *Cancer* 45(1) (1980): 51-6.

Ghent W.R., Eskin B.A., et al. "Iodine replacement in fibrocystic disease of the breast." *Canadian Journal of Surgery* 36(5) (1993): 453-60.

Giani C., Fierabracci P., et al. "Relationship between breast cancer and thyroid disease: relevance of autoimmune thyroid disorders in breast malignancy." *Journal of Clinical Endocrinology Metabolism* 81(3) (1996): 990-4.

Girdler S.S., Hinderliter A.L., et al. "Transdermal versus oral estrogen in postmenopausal smokers: hemodynamic and endothelial effects." *Obstetrics and Gynecology* 103(1) (2004): 169-80.

Goodman J.E., Lavigne J.A., et al. "COMT genotype, micronutrients in the folate metabolic pathway and breast cancer risk." *Carcinogenesis* 22(10) (2001): 1661-5.

Goodman M.T., McDuffie K., et al. "Association of methylenetetrahydrofolate reductase polymorphism C677T and dietary folate with the risk of cervical dysplasia." *Cancer Epidemiology Biomarkers and Prevention* 10(12) (2001): 1275-80.

Goodman M.T., McDuffie K., et al. "Case-control study of ovarian cancer and polymorphisms in genes involved in catecholestrogen formation and metabolism." *Cancer Epidemiology Biomarkers and Prevention* 10(3) (2001): 209-16.

Goodwin P.J., Ennis M., et al. "Fasting insulin and outcome in early-stage breast cancer: results of a prospective cohort study." *Journal of Clinical Oncology* 20(1) (2002): 42-51.

Gregus Z., Gyurasics A., et al. "Effects of arsenic-, platinum-, and gold-containing drugs on the disposition of exogenous selenium in rats." *Toxicological Sciences* 57(1) (2000): 22-31.

Grodstein F., Stampfer M.J. "Postmenopausal hormone therapy and mortality." *New England Journal of Medicine* 336(25) (1997): 1769-75.

Guarner F., Malagalada J.R. "Gut flora in health and disease." *Lancet* 361(9371) (2003): 512-9.

Gupta D., Lis C.G., et al. "Bioelectrical impedance phase angle as a prognostic indicator in advanced pancreatic cancer." *British Journal of Nutrition* Dec 92(6) (2004): 957-62.

Gupta K., Krishnaswamy G., et al. "Insulin: a novel factor in carcinogenesis." *American Journal of the Medical Sciences* 323(3) (2002): 140-5.

Gurates B., Bulun S.E., et al. "Endometriosis: the ultimate hormonal disease." *Seminars in Reproductive Medicine* 21(2) (2003): 125-34.

Hachey D.L., Dawling S., et al. "Sequential action of phase I and II enzymes cytochrome p450 1B1 and glutathione S-transferase P1 in mammary estrogen metabolism." *Cancer Research* 63(23) (2003): 8492-9.

Haggans C.J., Hutchins A.M., et al. "Effect of flaxseed consumption on urinary estrogen metabolites in postmenopausal women." *Nutrition and Cancer* 33(2) (1999): 188-95.

Hakimuddin F., Paliyath G., et al. "Selective cytotoxicity of a red grape wine flavonoid fraction against MCF-7 cells." *Breast Cancer Research and Treatment* 85(1) (2004): 65-79.

Hall D.C. "Nutritional influences on estrogen metabolism." *Applied Nutritional Science Reports* (2001): 1-8.

Han W., Kang D., et al. "Associations between breast cancer susceptibility gene polymorphisms and clinicopathological features." *Clinical Cancer Research* 10(1 Part 1) (2004): 124-30.

Hanna I.H., Dawling S., et al. "Cytochrome P450 1B1 (CYP1B1) pharmacogenetics: association of polymorphisms with functional differences in estrogen hydroxylation activity." *Cancer Research* 60(13) (2000): 3440-4.

Harvey J.A., Bovbjerg V.E. "Quantitative assessment of mammographic breast density: relationship with breast cancer risk." *Radiology* 230(1) (2004): 29-41.

Heerdt A.S., Young C.W., et al. "Calcium glucarate as a chemopreventive agent in breast cancer." *Israel Journal of Medical Science* 31(2-3) (1995): 101-5.

Helzlsouer K.J., Selmin O., et al. "Association between glutathione S-transferase M1, P1, and T1 genetic polymorphisms and development of breast cancer." *Journal of the National Cancer Institute* 90(7) (1998): 512-8.

Henson M.C., Chedrese P.J. "Endocrine disruption by cadmium, a common environmental toxicant with paradoxical effects on reproduction." *Experimental Biology and Medicine (Maywood)* 229(5) (2004): 383-92.

Herrmann S., Seidelin M., et al. "Indolo[3,2-b]carbazole inhibits gap junctional intercellular communication in rat primary hepatocytes and acts as a potential tumor promoter." *Carcinogenesis* 23(11) (2002): 1861-8.

Heidi K.B., Jack H.W. "The effects of a 20-week exercise training program on resting metabolic rate in previously sedentary, moderately obese women." *International Journal of Sport Nutrition and Exercise Metabolism* 11(1) (2001): 15-31.

Hinz, Marty. Personal communication. NeuroResearch Clinics Seminars. 2004.

Hodges L.C., Bergerson J.S., et al. "Estrogenic effects of organochlorine pesticides on uterine leiomyoma cells *in vitro*." *Toxicological Sciences* 54(2) (2000): 355-64.

Hofseth L.J., Raafat A.M., et al. "Hormone replacement therapy with estrogen or estrogen plus medroxyprogesterone acetate is associated with increased epithelial proliferation in the postmenopausal breast." *Journal of Clinical Endocrinology and Metabolism* 84(12) (1999): 4559-65.

Holick, Michael, and Mark Jenkins. *The UV Advantage.* ibooks, 2003.

Hollowell J.E., Staehling N.W., et al. "Iodine nutrition in the United States. Trends and public health implications: iodine excretion data from National Health and Nutrition Examination Surveys I and III (1971-1974 and 1988-1994)." *Journal of Clinical Endocrinology and Metabolism* 83(10) (1998): 3401-8.

von Holtz R.L., Fink C.S., et al. "beta-Sitosterol activates the sphingomyelin cycle and induces apoptosis in LNCaP human prostate cancer cells." *Nutrition and Cancer* 32(1) (1998): 8-12.

Hung L.M., Chen J.K., et al. "Cardioprotective effect of resveratrol, a natural antioxidant derived from grapes." *Cardiovascular Research* 47(3) (2000): 549-55.

John E.M., Dreon D.M., et al. "Residential sunlight exposure is associated with a decrease risk of prostate cancer." *Journal of Steroid Biochemistry and Molecular Biology* 89-90(1-5) (2004): 549-52.

John E.M., Schwartz G.G., et al. "Vitamin D and breast cancer risk: the NHANES I Epidemiologic follow-up study, 1971-1975 to 1992. National Health and Nutrition Examination Survey." *Cancer Epidemiology Biomarkers and Prevention* 8(5) (1999): 399-406.

Johnson M.D., Kenney N., et al. "Cadmium mimics the *in vivo* effects of estrogen in the uterus and mammary gland." *Nature Medicine* 9(8) (2003): 1081-4.

Kamel H.K., Maas D., et al. "Role of hormones in the pathogenesis and management of sarcopenia." *Drugs and Aging* 19(11) (2002): 865-77.

Kessler J.H. "The effect of supraphysiologic levels of iodine on patients with cyclic mastalgia." *Breast Journal* 10(4) (2004): 328-36.

Keyserlingk J.R., Ahlgren P.D., et al. "Functional infrared imaging of the breast." *IEEE Engineering in Medicine and Biology Magazine* 19(3) (2000): 30-41.

Kikuchi N., Urabe M., et al. "Atheroprotective effect of estriol and estrone sulfate on human vascular smooth muscle cells." *Journal of Steroid Biochemistry and Molecular Biology* 72(1-2) (2000): 71-8.

Kilbane M.T., Ajjan R.A., et al. "Tissue iodine content and serum-mediated 125I uptake-blocking activity in breast cancer." *Journal of Clinical Endocrinology and Metabolism* 85(3) (2000): 1245-50.

Koh K.K., Mincemoyer R., et al. "Effects of hormone-replacement therapy on fibrinolysis in postmenopausal women." *New England Journal of Medicine* 336(10) (1997): 683-90.

Kolata G. B. "!Kung hunter-gatherers: feminism, diet and birth control." *Science* 185 (1974): 932-4.

Kumar A.P., Garcia G.E., et al. "2-methoxyestradiol blocks cell-cycle progression at G(2)/M phase and inhibits growth of human prostate cancer cells." *Molecular Carcinogenesis* 31(3) (2001): 111-24.

Labrie F., Luu-The V., et al. "Endocrine and intracrine sources of androgens in women: inhibition of breast cancer and other roles of androgens and their precursor dehydroepiandrosterone." *Endocrine Reviews* 24(2) (2003): 152-82.

Larsson S.C., Kumlin M., et al. "Dietary long-chain n-3 fatty acids for the prevention of cancer: a review of potential mechanisms." *American Journal of Clinical Nutrition* 79(6) (2004): 935-45.

Lauritzen C. "Results of a 5 years prospective study of estriol succinate treatment in patients with climacteric complaints." *Hormone and Metabolic Research* 19(11) (1987): 579-84.

Lewis J.G., McGill H., et al. "Caution on the use of saliva measurements to monitor absorption of progesterone from transdermal creams in postmenopausal women." *Maturitas* 41(1) (2002): 1-6.

Li D.N., Seidel A., et al. "Polymorphisms in P450 CYP1B1 affect the conversion of estradiol to the potentially carcinogenic metabolite 4-hydroxyestradiol." *Pharmacogenetics* 10(4) (2000): 343-53.

de Lignieres B., deVathaire F., et al. "Combined hormone replacement therapy and risk of breast cancer in a French cohort study of 3175 women." *Climateric* 5(4) (2002): 332-40.

Lillberg K., Verkasalo P.K., et al. "Stressful life events and risk of breast cancer in 10,808 women: a cohort study." *American Journal of Epidemiology* 157(5) (2003): 415-23.

Liu R.H., Liu J., et al. "Apples prevent mammary tumors in rats." *Journal of Agricultural and Food Chemistry* 53(6) (2005): 2341-3.

Liu Z.J., Zhu B.T. "Concentration-dependent mitogenic and antiproliferative actions of 2-methoxyestradiol in estrogen receptor-positive human breast cancer cells." *Journal of Steroid Biochemistry and Molecular Biology* 88(3) (2004): 265-75.

Longscope C. "Estriol production and metabolism in normal women." *Journal of Steroid Biochemistry* 20(4B) (1984): 959-62.

Lord R.S., Bongiovanni B., et al. "Estrogen metabolism and the diet-cancer connection: rationale for assessing the ratio of urinary hydroxylated estrogen metabolites." *Alternative Medicine Review* 7(2) (2002): 112-29.

Lundstrom E., Wilczek B., et al. "Mammographic breast density during hormone replacement therapy: effects of continuous combination, unopposed transdermal and low-potency estrogen regimens." *Climateric* 4(1) (2001): 42-8.

Luukkainen T. "Issues to debate on the Women's Health Initiative: failure of estrogen plus progestin therapy for prevention of breast cancer risk." *Human Reproduction* 18(8) (2003): 1559-61.

Ma X., Yang Q., et al. "Promoter methylation regulates cyclooxygenase expression in breast cancer." *Breast Cancer Research* 6(4) (2004): R316-21.

Mady E.A., Ramadan E.E., et al. "Sex steroid hormones in serum and tissue of benign and malignant breast tumor patients." *Disease Markers* 16(3-4) (2001): 151-7.

Marchioli R., Barzi F., et al. "Early protection against sudden death by n-3 polyunsaturated fatty acids after myocardial infarction: time-course analysis of the results of the Gruppo Italiano per lo Studio della Sopravvivenza nell'Infarto Miocardico (GISSI)-Prevenzione." *Circulation* 105(16) (2002): 1897-1903.

Matthews C.E., Fowke J.H., et al. "Physical activity, body size, and estrogen metabolism in women." *Cancer Causes and Control* 15(5) (2004): 473-81.

McCullough L.D., Hurn P.D. "Estrogen and ischemic neuroprotection: an integrated view." *Trends in Endocrinology and Metabolism* 14(5) (2003): 228-35.

McFadyen M.C., Cruickshank M.E., et al. "Cytochrome P450 CYP1B1 over-expression in primary and metastatic ovarian cancer." *British Journal of Cancer* 85(2) (2001): 242-6.

McGrath M., Hankinson S.E., et al. "Cytochrome P450 1B1 and catechol-O-methyltransferase polymorphisms and endometrial cancer susceptibility." *Carcinogenesis* 25(4) (2004): 559-65.

McLachlan J.A. "Environmental signaling: what embryos and evolution teach us about endocrine disrupting chemicals." *Endocrine Reviews* 22(3) (2001): 319-41.

Melamed M., Castano E., et al. "Molecular and kinetic basis for the mixed agonist/antagonist activity of estriol." *Molecular Endocrinology* 11(12) (1997): 1868-78.

Michels K.B., Holmberg L., et al. "Coffee, tea, and caffeine consumption and breast cancer incidence in a cohort of Swedish women." *Annals of Epidemiology* 12(1) (2002): 21-6.

Minton J.P., Walaszek Z., et al. "beta-glucuronidase levels in patients with fibrocystic breast disease." *Breast Cancer Research and Treatment* 8(3) (1986): 217-22.

Mitrunen K., Hirvonen A. "Molecular epidemiology of sporadic breast cancer. The role of polymorphic genes involved in oestrogen biosynthesis and metabolism." *Mutation Research* 544(1) (2003): 9-41.

Modugno F., Knoll C., et al. "A potential role for the estrogen-metabolizing cytochrome P450 enzymes in human breast carcinogenesis." *Breast Cancer Research and Treatment* 82(3) (2003): 191-7.

Moffat S.D., Zonderman A.B., et al. "Free testosterone and risk for Alzheimer disease in older men." *Neurology* 62(2) (2004): 188-93.

Mohr P.E., Wang D.Y., et al. "Serum progesterone and prognosis in operable breast cancer." *British Journal of Cancer* 73(12) (1996): 1552-5.

Mor G., Yue W., et al. "Macrophages, estrogen and the micro-environment of breast cancer." *Journal of Steroid Biochemistry and Molecular Biology* 67(5-6) (1998): 403-11.

Morales A. "Androgen replacement therapy and prostate safety." *European Urology* 41(2) (2002): 113-20.

Mueck A.O., Seeger H., et al. "Chemotherapy of breast cancer-additive anticancerogenic effects by 2-methoxyestradiol?" *Life Sciences* 75(10) (2004): 1205-10.

Mueck A.O., Seeger H., et al. "Comparison of the proliferative effects of estradiol and conjugated equine estrogens on human breast cancer cells and impact of continuous combined progestogen addition." *Climateric* 6(3) (2003): 221-7.

Mueck A.O., Seeger H., et al. "Impact of hormone replacement therapy on endogenous estradiol metabolism in postmenopausal women." *Maturitas* 43(2) (2002): 87-93.

Mueck A.O., Seeger H. "Smoking, estradiol metabolism and hormone replacement therapy." *Arzneimittelforschung* 53(1) (2003): 1-11.

Mutaku J.F., Poma J.F., et al. "Cell necrosis and apoptosis are differentially regulated during goiter development and iodine-induced involution." *Journal of Endocrinology* 172(2) (2002): 375-86.

Muti P., Bradlow H.L., et al. "Estrogen metabolism and risk of breast cancer: a prospective study of the 2:16alpha-hydroxyestrone ratio in premenopausal and postmenopausal women." *Epidemiology* 11(6) (2000): 635-40.

Nash D., Magdler L., et al. "Blood lead, blood pressure, and hypertension in perimenopausal and postmenopausal women." *Journal of the American Medical Association* 289(12) (2003): 1523-32.

Needleman S.W., Stump D.C., et al. "Catechol estrogens and thrombosis: lack of a direct effect of 2-hydroxyestradiol on platelets." *Contraception* 25(2) (1982): 185-9.

Negri S., Bonetti F., et al. "Preoperative diagnostic accuracy of fine-needle aspiration in the management of breast lesions: comparison of specificity and sensitivity with clinical examination, mammography, echography, and thermography in 249 patients." *Diagnostic Cytopathology* 11(1) (1994): 4-8.

Ng E., Sudharson N.M. "Computer simulation in conjunction with medical thermography as an adjunct tool for early detection of breast cancer." *BMC Cancer* 4(1) (2004): 17.

O'Brien S.N., Anandjiwala J., et al. "Differences in the estrogen content of breast adipose tissue in women by menopausal status and hormonal use." *Obstetrics and Gynecology* 90(2) (1997): 244-8.

Oger E., Alhenc-Gelas M., et al. "Differential effects of oral and transdermal estrogen/progesterone regimens on sensitivity to activated protein C among postmenopausal women: a randomized trial." *Arteriosclerosis Thrombosis Vascular Biology* 23(9) (2003): 1671-6.

Olsen A.H., Njor S.H., et al. "Breast cancer mortality in Copenhagen after introduction of mammography screening: cohort study." *BMJ* 330(7485) (2005): 220.

Palomba S., Sena T., et al. "Transdermal hormone replacement therapy in postmenopausal women with uterine leiomyoma." *Obstetrics and Gynecology* 98(6) (2001): 1053-8.

Parl, Fritz F. *Estrogens, Estrogen Receptor, and Breast Cancer.* IOS Press, 2000.

Pasqualini J.R., Chetrite G.S. "Recent insight on the control of enzymes involved in estrogen formation and transformation in human breast cancer." *Journal of Steroid Biochemistry and Molecular Biology* 93(2-5) (2005): 221-36.

Pascqualini J.R., Schatz B., et al. "Recent data on estrogen sulfatases and sulfotransferases activities in human breast cancer." *Journal of Steroid Biochemistry and Molecular Biology* 41(3-8) (1992): 323-9.

Peter G.F., Chun Y.J., et al. "Cytochrome P450 1B1: a target for inhibition in anticarcinogenesis strategies." *Mutation Research* 1523-524 (2003): 73-82.

Pfeilschifter J., Koditz R., et al. "Changes in proinflammatory cytokine activity after menopause." *Endocrine Review* 23(1) (2002): 90-119.

Phillips G.B., Pinkernell B.H., et al. "Are major risk factors for myocardial infarction the major predictors of degree of coronary artery disease in men?" *Metabolism* 53(3) (2003): 324-9.

Pischinger, Alfred. *Matrix and Matrix Regulation. Basis for a Holistic Theory in Medicine.* Medicina Biologica, 1991.

Portier C.J. "Endocrine dismodulation and cancer." *Neuro Endocrinology Letters* 23 Supplement 2 (2002): 43-7.

Potter G.A., Patterson L.H., et al. "The cancer preventative agent resveratrol is converted to the anticancer agent piceatannol by the cytochrome P450 enzyme CYP1B1." *British Journal of Cancer* 86(5) (2002): 774-8.

Prior J.C. "Progesterone as a bone-trophic hormone." *Endocrine Reviews* 11(2) (1990): 386-98.

Raju U., Sepkovic D.W., et al. "Estrone and estradiol metabolism *in vivo* in human breast cysts." *Steroids* 65(12) (2000): 883-8.

Reiss, Uzzi, Martin Zucker. *Natural Hormonal Balance for Women.* Atria, 2002.

Rogan E.G., Badawi A.F., et al. "Relative imbalances in estrogen metabolism and conjugation in breast tissue of women with carcinoma: potential biomarkers of susceptibility to cancer." *Carcinogenesis* 24(4) (2003): 697-702.

Rose D.P., Komninou D., et al. "Obesity, adipocytokines, and insulin resistance in breast cancer." *Obesity Reviews* 5(3) (2004): 153-165.

Ross J.A., Kasum C.M. "Dietary flavonoids: bioavailability, metabolic effects, and safety." *Annual Review of Nutrition* 22 (2002): 19-34.

Ross S.A. "Diet and DNA methylation interactions in cancer prevention." *Annals of the New York Academy of Sciences* 983 (2002): 197-207.

Rowland I., Wiseman T., et al. "Metabolism of oestrogens and phytoestrogens: role of the gut microflora." *Biochemical Society Transactions* 27(2) (1999): 304-8.

Rylander-Rudqvist T., Wedren S., et al. "Cytochrome P450 1B1 gene polymorphisms and postmenopausal breast cancer risk." *Carcinogenesis* 24(9) (2003): 1533-9.

Saarinen N., Joshi S.C., et al. "No evidence for the *in vivo* activity of aromatase-inhibiting flavonoids." *Journal of Steroid Biochemistry and Molecular Biology* 78(3) (2001): 231-9.

Sadikovic B., Haines T.R., et al. "Chemically induced DNA hypomethylation in breast carcinoma cells detected by the amplification of intermethylated sites." *Breast Cancer Research* 6(4) (2004): R329-37.

Safe S., McDougal A. "Mechanism of action and development of selective aryl hydrocarbon receptor modulators for treatment of hormone-dependent cancers (Review)." *International Journal of Oncology* 20(6) (2002): 1123-8.

Saintot M., Malaveille C., et al. "Interactions between genetic polymorphism of cytochrome P450-1B1, sulfotransferase 1A1, catechol-O-methyltransferase and tobacco exposure in breast cancer risk." *International Journal of Cancer* 107(4) (2003): 652-7.

Saintot M., Malaveille C., et al. "Interaction between genetic polymorphism of cytochrome P450-1B1 and environmental pollutants in breast cancer risk." *European Journal of Cancer Prevention* 13(1) (2004): 83-6.

Sands R., Studd J. "Hormone replacement therapy for women after breast carcinoma." *Current Opinion in Obstetrics and Gynecology* 8(3) (1996): 216-20.

Sasaki M., Tanaka Y., et al. "CYP1B1 gene polymorphisms have higher risk for endometrial cancer, and positive correlations with estrogen receptor alpha and estrogen receptor beta expressions." *Cancer Research* 63(14) (2003): 3913-8.

Schaumberg D.A., Mendes F., et al. "Accumulated lead exposure and risk of age-related cataract in men." *Journal of the American Medical Association* 292(22) (2004): 2750-4.

Schernhammer E.S., Kang J.H., et al. "A prospective study of aspirin use and the risk of pancreatic cancer in women." *Journal of the National Cancer Institute* 96(1) (2004): 22-8.

Schiff I., Wentworth B., et al. "Effect of estriol administration on the hypogonadal woman." *Fertility and Sterility* 30(3) (1978): 278-82.

Schneider J., Huh M.M., et al. "Antiestrogen action of 2-hydroxy-estrone on MCF-7 human breast cancer cells." *Journal of Biological Chemistry* 259(8) (1984): 4840-5.

Schoeller D.A. "Bioelectrical impedance analysis. What does it measure?" *Annals of the New York Academy of Science* 904 (2000): 159-62.

Sears, Barry. *The Omega Rx Zone: The Miracle of the New High-Dose Fish Oil.* Regan Books, 2003.

Seeger H., Huober J., et al. "Inhibition of human breast cancer cell proliferation with estradiol metabolites is as effective as with tamoxifen." *Hormone and Metabolic Research* 36(5) (2004): 277-80.

Seeger H., Wallwiener D., et al. "Influence of stroma-derived growth factors on the estradiol-stimulated proliferation of human breast cancer cells." *European Journal of Gynaecological Oncology* 25(2) (2004): 175-7.

Sephton S.E., Sapolsky R.M., et al. "Diurnal cortisol rhythm as a predictor of breast cancer survival." *Journal of the National Cancer Institute* 92(12) (2000): 994-1000.

Sepkovic D.W., Bradlow H.L., et al. "Estrogen metabolite ratios and risk assessment of hormone-related cancers. Assay validation and prediction of cervical cancer risk." *Annals of the New York Academy of Sciences* 768 (1995): 312-6.

Shering S.G., Zbar A.P., et al. "Thyroid disorders and breast cancer." *European Journal of Cancer Prevention* 5(6) (1996): 504-6.

Sherwin B.B. "Estrogen and cognitive functioning in women." *Endocrine Review* 24(2) (2003): 133-51.

Shippen, Eugene, William Fryer. *The Testosterone Syndrome.* M. Evans and Company, Inc., 2001.

Short R.V. "Definition of the problem: The evolution of human reproduction." *Proceeding of the Royal Society London B* 195 (1976): 3-24.

Short K.R., Nair K.S. "Muscle protein metabolism and the sarcopenia of aging." *International Journal of Sport Nutrition and Exercise Metabolism* 11 Supplement (2001): S119-27.

Shozu M., Murakami K., et al. "Aromatase and leiomyoma of the uterus." *Seminars in Reproductive Medicine* 22(1) (2004): 51-60.

Sieri S., Krogh V., et al. "Dietary patterns and risk of breast cancer in the ORDET cohort." *Cancer Epidemiology Biomarkers and Prevention* 13(4) (2004): 562-72.

Simopoulos A.P. "Importance of the ratio of omega-6/omega-3 essential fatty acids." *Biomedicine and Pharmacotherapy* 56(8) (2002): 365-79.

Singletary K., MacDonald C., et al. "Inhibition by rosemary and carnosol of 7,12-dimethylbenz[a]anthracene (DMBA)-induced rat mammary tumorigenesis and *in vivo* DMBA-DNA adduct formation." *Cancer Letters* 104(1) (1996): 43-8.

Sitruk-Ware R, Seradour B, et al. "Treatment of benign breast diseases by progesterone applied topically." In: *Percutaneous Absorption of Steroids.* New York, NY: Academic Press, 1980: 219-229.

Slavin J. "Why whole grains are protective: biological mechanisms." *Proceedings of the Nutrition Society* 62(1) (2003): 129-34.

Smyth P.P. "The thyroid, iodine and breast cancer." *Breast Cancer Research* 5(5) (2003): 235-8.

Somboonporn W., Davis S.R., et al. "Testosterone effects on the breast: implications for testosterone therapy for women." *Endocrine Reviews* 25(3) (2004): 374-88.

Song R.X., Mor G., et al. "Effect of long-term estrogen deprivation on apoptotic responses of breast cancer cells to 17β-estradiol." *Journal of the National Cancer Institute* 93(22) (2001): 1714-23.

Sonnenschein C., Soto A.M. "Somatic mutation theory of carcinogenesis: why it should be dropped and replaced." *Molecular Carcinogenesis* 29(4) (2000): 205-11.

Soto A.M., Sonnenschein C. "The two faces of Janus: Sex steroids as mediators of both cell proliferation and cell death." *Journal of the National Cancer Institute* 93(22) (2001): 1673-5.

Speroff, Leon, Robert H. Glass, et al. *Clinical Gynecologic Endocrinology and Infertility. Sixth Edition.* Lippincott Williams and Wilkins, 1999.

Spink D.C., Zhang F., et al. "Metabolism of equilenin in MCF-7 and MDA-MB-231 human breast cancer cells." *Chemical Research in Toxicology* 14(5) (2001): 572-81.

Spitzweg C., Harrington K.J., et al. "Clinical review 132: The sodium iodide symporter and its potential role in cancer therapy." *Journal of Clinical Endocrinology and Metabolism* 86(7)(2001): 3327-35.

Stadel B.V. "Dietary iodine and risk of breast, endometrial, and ovarian cancer." *Lancet* 1(7965) (1976): 890-1.

Starek A. "Estrogens and organochlorine xenoestrogens and breast cancer risk." *International Journal of Occupational Medicine and Environmental Health* 16(2) (2003): 113-24.

Stejskal V.D., Danersund A., et al. "Metal-specific lymphocytes: biomarkers of sensitivity in man." *Neuro Endocrinology Letters* 20(5) (1999): 289-98.

Stewart J.R., Artime M.C., et al. "Resveratrol: a candidate nutritional substance for prostate cancer prevention." *Journal of Nutrition* 133(7 Supplement) (2003): 2440S-2443S.

Suganuma M., Okabe S., et al. "Green tea and cancer chemoprevention." *Mutation Research* 428(1-2) (1999): 339-44.

Sumino H., Ichikawa S., et al. "Hormone Replacement therapy decreases insulin resistance and lipid metabolism in Japanese postmenopausal women with impaired and normal glucose tolerance." *Hormone Research* 60(3) (2003): 134-42.

Surh Y. "Molecular mechanisms of chemopreventive effects of selected dietary and medicinal phenolic substances." *Mutation Research* 428(1-2) (1999): 305-27.

Suzuki T., Miki Y., et al. "Steroid sulfatase and estrogen sulfotransferase in normal human tissue and breast carcinoma." *Journal of Steroid Biochemistry and Molecular Biology* 86(3-5) (2003): 449-54.

Teepker M., Anthes N., et al. "2-OH-estradiol, an endogenous hormone with neuroprotective functions." *Journal of Psychiatric Research* 37(6) (2003): 517-23.

Telang N.T., Bradlow H.L., et al. "Molecular and endocrine biomarkers in non-involved breast: relevance to cancer chemoprevention." *Journal of Cellular Biochemistry* 16G (1992): 161-9.

Tempfer C.B., Schneeberger C., et al. "Applications of polymorphisms and pharmacogenomics in obstetrics and gynecology." *Pharmacogenomics* 5(1) (2004): 57-65.

Thier R., Bruning T., et al. "Markers of genetic susceptibility in human environmental hygiene and toxicology: the role of selected CYP, NAT and GST genes." *International Journal of Hygiene and Environmental Health* 206(3) (2003): 148-71.

Thomas T., Rhodin J., et al. "Progestins initiate adverse events of menopausal estrogen therapy." *Climateric* 6(4) (2003): 293-301.

Toy J.L., Davies J.A., et al. "The effects of long-term therapy with oestriol succinate on the haemostatic mechanism in postmenopausal women." *British Journal of Obstetrics and Gynecology* 85(5) (1978): 363-6.

Tulchinsky D., Hobel C.J., et al. "Plasma estrone, estradiol, estriol, progesterone, and 17-hydroxyprogesterone in human pregnancy." *American Journal of Obstetrics and Gynecology* 112(8) (1972): 1095-100.

Tworoger S.S., Chuback J., et al. "Association of CYP17, CYP19, CYP1B1, and COMT polymorphisms with serum and urinary sex hormone concentrations in postmenopausal women." *Cancer Epidemiology Biomarkers and Prevention* 13(1) (2004): 94-101.

Ursin G., London S., et al. "A pilot study of urinary estrogen metabolites (16alpha-OHE1 and 2-OHE1) in postmenopausal women with and without breast cancer." *Environmental Health Perspectives* 105 Supplement 3 (1997): 601-5.

Van Niekerk W. A. "Cervical cytological abnormalities caused by folic acid deficiency." *Acta Cytologica* 10 (1966): 67-73.

Velicer C.M., Heckbert S.R., et al. "Antibiotic use in relation to the risk of breast cancer." *Journal of the American Medical Association* 291(7) (2004): 827-35.

Velicer C.M., Lampe J.W., et al. "Hypothesis: is antibiotic use associated with breast cancer?" *Cancer Causes and Control* 14(8) (2003): 739- 47.

Venturi S. "Is there a role for iodine in breast diseases?" *Breast* 10(5) (2001): 379-82.

Vermeulen A., Deslypere J.P., et al. "Aromatase, 17 beta-hydroxysteroid dehydrogenase and intratissular sex hormone concentrations in cancerous and normal glandular breast tissue in postmenopausal women." *European Journal of Cancer and Clinical Oncology* 22(4) (1986): 515-25.

Vorderstrasse B.A., Fenton S.E. "A novel effect of dioxin: exposure during pregnancy severely impairs mammary gland differentiation." *Toxicological Sciences* 78(2) (2004): 248-57.

Wakatsuki A., Okatani Y., et al. "Effect of medroxyprogesterone acetate on endothelium dependent vasodilation in postmenopausal women receiving estrogen." *Circulation* 104(15) (2001): 1773-8.

Walaszek Z., Szemraj J., et al. "Metabolism, uptake, and excretion of a D-glucaric acid salt and its potential in cancer prevention." *Cancer Detection and Prevention* 21(2) (1997): 178-90.

Walaszek Z., Hanausek-Walaszek M., et al. "Dietary glucarate as anti-promoter of 7,12-dimethylbenz[a]anthracene-induced mammary tumorigenesis." *Carcinogenesis* 7(9) (1986): 1463-6.

Wallace J.M. "Nutritional and botanical modulation of the inflammatory cascade -- eicosanoids, cyclooxygenases, and lipoxygenases -- as an adjunct in cancer therapy." *Integrative Cancer Therapies* 1(1) (2002): 7-37.

Warmuth M.A., Sutton L.M., et al. "A review of hereditary breast cancer: from screening to risk factor modification." *American Journal of Medicine* 102(4) (1997): 407-15.

Warner M., Eskenazi B., et al. "Serum dioxin concentrations and breast cancer risk in the Seveso Women's Health Study." *Environmental Health Perspectives* 110(7) (2002): 625-8.

Webb P.M., Byrne C., et al. "A prospective study of diet and benign breast disease." *Cancer Epidemiology Biomarkers and Prevention* 13(7) (2004): 1106-13.

Wiebe J.P., Lewis M.J., et al. "The role of progesterone metabolites in breast cancer: potential for new diagnostics and therapeutics." *Journal of Steroid Biochemistry and Molecular Biology* 93(2-5) (2005): 201-8.

Wietzke J.A., Welsh J. "Phytoestrogen regulation of a vitamin D3 receptor promoter and 1,25-dihydroxyvitamin D3 actions in human breast cancer cells." *Journal of Steroid Biochemistry and Molecular Biology* 84(2-3) (2003): 149-57.

Willett, Walter. *Eat, Drink, and Be Healthy.* Free Press, 2001.

Williams K.L., Phillips B.H., et al. "Thermography in screening for breast cancer." *Journal Epidemiology and Community Health* 44(2) (1990): 112-3.

Women's Health Initiative, www.nhlbi.nih.gov/whi/.

Wren B.G. "Hormonal replacement therapy and breast cancer." *European Menopause Journal* 2(4) (1995): 13-19.

Wren B.G., McFarland K., et al. "Effect of sequential transdermal progesterone cream on endometrium, bleeding pattern, and plasma progesterone and salivary progesterone levels in postmenopausal women." *Climacteric* 3(3) (2000): 153-4.

Wren B.G. "The breast and the menopause." *Bailliere's Clinical Obstetrics and Gynaecology* 10(3) (1996): 433-47.

Wright T., McGechan A. "Breast cancer: new technologies for risk assessment and diagnosis." *Molecular Diagnosis* 7(1) (2003): 49-55.

Zacharia L.C., Gogos J.A., et al. "Methoxyestradiols mediate the antimitogenic effects of 17beta-estradiol: direct evidence from catechol-O-methyltransferase-knockout mice." *Circulation* 108(24) (2003): 2974-8.

Zacharia L.C., Piche C.A., et al. "2-hydroxyestradiol is a prodrug of 2-methoxyestradiol." *Journal of Pharmacology and Experimental Therapy* 309(3) (2004): 1093-7.

Zandi P.P., Carlson M.C., et al. "Hormone replacement therapy and incidence of Alzheimer disease in older women: the Cache County Study." *Journal of the American Medical Association* 288(17) (2002): 2123-9.

Zeligs M.A. "Diet and estrogen status: the cruciferous connection." *Journal of Medicinal Food* 1(2) (1998): 67-82.

Zhang F., Chen Y., et al. "The major metabolite of equilin, 4-hydroxyequilin, autoxidizes to an o-quinone which isomerizes to the potent cytotoxin 4-hydroxyequilenin-o-quinone." *Chemical Research in Toxicology* 12(2) (1999): 204-13.

Zhang S.M., Willett W., et al. "Plasma folate, vitamin B6, vitamin B12, homocysteine, and risk of breast cancer." *Journal of the National Cancer Institute* 95(5) (2003): 373-80.

Zhang Y., Jayaprakasam B., et al. "Insulin secretion and cyclooxygenase enzyme inhibition by cabernet sauvignon grape skin compounds." *Journal of Agricultural and Food Chemistry* 52(2) (2004): 228-33.

Zheng W., Gustafson D.R., et al. "Well-done meat intake and the risk of breast cancer." *Journal of the National Cancer Institute* 90(22) (1998): 1724-9.

Zheng W., Jin F., et al. "Epidemiological study of urinary 6 beta-hydroxycortisol to cortisol ratios and breast cancer risk." *Cancer Epidemiology Biomarkers and Prevention* 10(3) (2001): 237-42.

Zheng W., Xie D.W., et al. "Genetic polymorphisms of cytochrome P450-1B1 and risk of breast cancer." *Cancer Epidemiology Biomarkers and Prevention* 9(2) (2000): 147-50.

Zhu B.T., Conney A.H. "Is 2-methoxyestradiol an endogenous estrogen metabolite that inhibits mammary carcinogenesis?" *Cancer Research* 58(11) (1998): 2269-77.

Zhu B.T. "Medical hypothesis: hyperhomocysteinemia is a risk factor for estrogen-induced hormonal cancer." *International Journal of Oncology* 22(3) (2003): 499-508.

Zhuang H., Kim Y.S., et al. "Potential mechanism by which resveratrol, a red wine constituent, protects neurons." *Annals of the New York Academy of Sciences* 993 (2003): 276-86.

Zumoff B. "Hormonal profiles in women with breast cancer." *Obstetrics and Gynecology Clinics of North America* 21(4) (1994): 751-72.

GLOSSARY

2-hydroxyestrogen (2OH): a breakdown product of estradiol that upon being methylated kills breast cancer cells. The enzyme CYP1A1 facilitates the formation of the 2OH estrogens, especially in the presence of the nutrient diindolylmethane.

4-hydroxyestrogens (4OH): is a downstream metabolite of estradiol. CYPIBI is the enzyme that facilitates its formation in the breast cell. 4OH estrogens are very damaging to the DNA of breast cells and can initiate cancer formation.

16α-hydroxyestrogen (16OH): is a downstream metabolite of estrone that is formed mainly in the liver. Elevated levels of 16OH estrogens like estradiol can induce excessive division of breast cells.

17β-hydroxysteroid dehydrogenase (17β-HSD): a family of enzymes that ultimately control the amount of estrogen that is formed within cells, particularly those of the breast and fat.

Acid: a hydrogen ion (protons) donor. An acid reacts with metal to form a salt, neutralizes bases, and turns litmus paper red. The pH of an acid is less than seven.

Adaptation: is the body's ability to undergo physiologic or behavioral changes in response to both intrinsic and extrinsic challenges. Loss of this ability results in accelerated aging. Adaptation is important to evolutionary biology since it increases survivability and reproductive capability of the organism.

Addison's disease: is a rare, potentially life-threatening hypofunctioning of the adrenal glands. It is listed as a "primary" failure because the glands themselves have ceased to produce cortisol, aldosterone, and other adrenal hormones.

Adrenal glands: Two pyramid-shaped glands located atop the kidneys, which secrete DHEA, cortisol, aldosterone, and adrenaline. The adrenals also secrete smaller amounts of progesterone, estrone, and estradiol. These glands regulate many vital functions including blood pressure, energy metabolism, and immune response. Chronic stress has detrimental effects on adrenal gland function.

Adrenaline (epinephrine): is a neurotransmitter released by the adrenal gland in response to stress.

Agonist: refers to a drug or compound that has the opposite effect of an antagonist. The agonist promotes a chemical reaction upon binding to another molecule's cell receptor. For example, in the absence of estradiol, soy (as an agonist) can bind to the estrogen receptor and initiate estrogen-driven cell reactions.

Aldosterone: is a hormone secreted by the adrenal glands that causes the kidney to retain sodium while eliminating potassium. This is an important determinant of blood pressure.

Alkaline: is the opposite of acid and has a pH greater than seven.

Alveolus: is a sac located within the breast that is lined by milk-producing cells. The alveolus empties the milk into a duct, where it is carried to the nipple.

Alzheimer's disease: A chronic disease of aging that involves the death of brain cells and is noted to worsen with time. Symptoms include memory loss, confusion, and a decline in physical abilities. Estrogen deficiency has been implicated as a predisposing factor in Alzheimer's.

Amalgam: is the "silver filling" used by dentists to fill the cavity left by tooth decay. Amalgams most often consist of 50 percent mercury, 35 percent silver, and 15 percent tin along with other metals. These metals, especially mercury, can leach into you tissues, which among other things can poison the immune system.

Anastrozole (Arimidex): is a pharmaceutical drug, which blocks the production of estradiol by inhibition of the enzyme aromatase. Arimidex is used in the treatment of breast cancer.

Androgens: From the Greek *andros* denoting male-like. Androgens are hormones that include testosterone and DHEA, which are important in sex drive, muscle development, sense of well-being, and energy. They are vital to the health of both women and men.

Andropause: is a syndrome in men that is associated with a decline in hormones, especially that of testosterone. Symptoms include: depression, fatigue, decreased sex drive, erectile dysfunction, decreased strength and muscle mass, and a decline in cognitive function. Also known as male menopause or viropause.

Androstenedione: An androgenic hormone, which can be converted into testosterone or estrogen.

Antibiotics: substances that are capable of inhibiting or killing bacteria. Antibiotics are generally produced by microorganisms and fungi. Examples are penicillin, streptomycin, and tetracycline.

Antagonist: refers to a specific drug or compound that binds to a cell receptor, blocking other molecules from binding. Antagonists inactivate the receptor's ability to initiate a specific chemical reaction. Soy (as an antagonist) can bind to the estradiol breast cell receptor, which prevents estradiol from initiating cell division.

Antioxidant: Any substance that quenches free radicals by electrical neutralization. Antioxidants such as vitamin E and vitamin C prevent DNA damage, which slows the aging process and decreases the chance of cancer formation.

Apoptosis: is programmed cell death.

Aromatase (CYP19): An intracellular enzyme that facilitates the conversion of testosterone to estradiol. Aromatase overactivity can lead to excessive intracellular levels of estradiol, increasing the risk of breast cancer. Red wine extract and drugs such as Femara block its action.

Basal body temperature (BBT): is determined by taking your temperature upon awakening. The thermometer should be placed in the axilla (under your arm) for seven to ten minutes. BBT indirectly measures both the energy expenditure at rest and the function of the thyroid.

Beta-glucuronidase: is an enzyme that reactivates estrogen by chemically freeing it from its deactivator molecule. This prevents estrogen from being removed from the body, causing it to recycle back into the bloodstream, which can result in excess levels.

Bio-identical hormones: are hormones that have the exact molecular structure as those made by your body. These are the preferred hormones for use in hormonal replacement therapy. Bio-identical hormones are also labeled as "natural" or "native" and are generally derived from vegetable sources such as soy or yams.

BRCA-1, 2: are tumor suppressor genes that if mutated can increase the potential for inheritable breast cancer.

Breast Care Pyramid: is program designed to help a woman avoid breast cancer while balancing her hormones, including estrogen. Following the pyramid suggestions sets the stage for healthy aging by protecting the heart, brain, and bones.

BreastSecure: consist of diindolylmethane, Ca D-glucarate, folic acid, folinic acid, and red wine extract suspended in an enhanced delivery system. BreastSecure acts to modulate estrogen levels in the breast cell and increase the production of the cancer-killing methylated 2OH estrogens. It also protects the prostate.

Butyrate: is an important food source for the cells that line the colon (colonocytes). Butyrate is derived from the fermentation of fiber by symbiotic bacteria. It has been reported to prevent colon cancer.

Calcium D-glucarate (Ca D-glucarate): is the long-acting calcium salt of D-glucaric acid. Glucaric acid is found in fruits and vegetables including apples, oranges, cauliflower, and broccoli. Ca D-glucarate prevents the enzyme beta-glucuronidase from reactivating estrogen. This recycled estrogen can lead to breast cell overstimulation and cancer.

Calorie: is the amount of heat or energy that is required to raise the temperature of one gram of water by one degree.

Carotenes: Part of the carotenoid nutrients found in the vitamin A family. Examples include beta-carotene, alpha-carotene, and gamma-carotene. Carotenes have a vitamin A activity of less than 10 percent.

C.A.N.: is a three-part program that restores intestinal function while removing toxins from the body: Cleanse — by removing any agent which undermines the integrity of the intestinal wall; Add — replace the health-promoting bacteria; and Nourish — provide the necessary supplements to help the good bacteria flourish while nurturing the intestinal cells (colonocytes).

Candida (yeast): is a yeast organism that is included within the larger category of fungi.

Cell differentiation: The process whereby a cell becomes physiologically specialized or mature.

Cellular matrix: is the biologic glue that holds cells together. It consists of a meshwork of high-polymer sugar-protein complexes.

Chelation: is derived from the Greek word *chela* — a claw. Chelation is a medical treatment involving the use of specialized molecules called chelators. The chelators bind to and inactivate toxins such as heavy metals.

Chelator: is a molecule whose strong electrical charge is able to bind to an atom such as a heavy metal. The ability to have a stronger attraction allows the chelator to inactivate and remove the atom from its surrounding tissue. Commonly used chelators include: Ethylenediaminetetraacetic acid (EDTA), dimercaptosuccinic acid (DMSA), and dimercaptopropane-sulfonic acid (DMPS).

Cholesterol: is the parent molecule for pregnenolone, estrogen, testosterone, progesterone, DHEA, and cortisol. Cholesterol, a major component of cell membranes, is made in the liver. Cholesterol also functions as an antioxidant. The inflammatory changes of aging can increase cholesterol levels, which can lead to its deposition and clogging of the blood vessels in the heart or brain.

Cortisol: A hormone produced by the adrenal gland, which is required for the conversion of carbohydrates, proteins, and fats into energy. Cortisol is a stress hormone, but also reduces inflammation.

Cushing's syndrome: arises from the excessive production of cortisol by the adrenal glands. Symptoms include being overweight, elevated blood glucose after carbohydrate-laden meals, and high blood pressure.

CYP1A1: is part of the cytochrome P450 enzyme family that is responsible for detoxification. CYP1A1 enzymes, located in breast cells, act upon estrone and estradiol to mainly produce the 2OH estrogens, which are capable of killing breast cancer cells. DIMN is an activator of CYP1A1.

CYP1B1: is a member of the cytochrome P450 family of detoxification enzymes. CYP1B1 activity increases the production of the DNA-damaging 4-OH estrogens.

Cytokines: are molecules that are mediators for producing anti-inflammatory or pro-inflammatory reactions in the body. Optimal health requires a balance of both types. Anti-inflammatory cytokines include interleukin-10 while pro-inflammatory cytokines include TNF-α and interleukin-1β.

D1, D2, D3: are three selenodeiodinase enzymes, which are responsible for the production of thyroid hormones. Selenium is a key element that is incorporated into the enzymatic structure. D1 is responsible for the production of T3 and is found mainly in the liver, kidney, thyroid gland, and pituitary gland. D2 is responsible for the majority of T3 production in the body and is present in most tissues. D3 is responsible for the breakdown of T3.

Detoxification: the removal of harmful substances, or toxins, from within your body.

DHEA (dehydroepiandrosterone): The most abundant hormone in the body and primarily made by the adrenal glands. DHEA is a prohormone that is converted into testosterone and even estrogen. It has been found to be protective of the breast, help with moods, balance the immune system, protect the heart, and control weight gain. Levels decline with aging.

DHEAS (dehydroepiandrosterone sulfate): When DHEA passes through the liver; a sulfate molecule is attached, which temporarily inactivates the hormone. This acts to form a reservoir of DHEA that the body can use as needed.

DHT (dihydrotestosterone): is a derivative of testosterone and is more potent, molecule for molecule. It protects the breast cell from cancer formation.

Diindolylmethane (DIMN): is derived from the acid breakdown of indole-3-carbinol in the stomach. DIMN interferes directly with breast cell division, preventing subsequent cancerous growths, and enhances the ability of CYP1A1 to metabolize breast estrogen into the cancer-killing 2OH estrogens.

Dihomo-gamma-linoleic acid (DGLA): is derived from the chemical conversion of the omega-6 gamma linolenic acid. DGLA can be potentially metabolized into the potent inflammatory arachidonic acid, but instead most studies have shown that it forms powerful anti-inflammatory hormones in the prostaglandin-one series. Increased levels of DGLA have been shown to be very beneficial in correcting chronic inflammatory conditions such as arthritis, eczema, and colitis.

DNA (deoxyribonucleic acid): are molecules that are the building blocks of life. They comprise your genetic code and consist of interlocking molecular bases that match up in specific patterns.

Ductal carcinoma in situ (DCIS): is the most common form of non-invasive breast cancer. It is found in the milk ducts and is generally detected by a mammogram.

EDTA (Ethylenediaminetetraacetic acid): see *chelator*.

Endometriosis: is a hormone-driven disease characterized by endometrial-like cells that line the abdominal cavity instead of the uterus. These cells bleed into the surrounding tissue and invoke an inflammatory response, characterized by pain and scarring.

Endometrium: The hormonally responsive inner lining of the uterus that is shed every month as a menstrual flow unless pregnancy ensues. Estrogens such as estradiol cause the endometrium to grow, while progesterone results in its maturation. A postmenopausal endometrium should be thin.

Enzyme: is a protein with a very specific role in promoting a chemical reaction that involves the rapid changing of a molecule into a different product. The enzyme does not get used up during this process.

Epidemiological: involves the study of the distribution and determinants of health-related states and events in populations.

Estradiol: is the most biologically active of the natural estrogens. During premenopause, it is primarily made by the ovaries, while in postmenopause, it is derived from the conversion of androstenedione in fat cells. Estradiol is an important hormone needed to delay the aging process in women and should be included in replacement therapy. Prolonged elevation of estradiol, however, can lead to excess breast cell division.

Estriol: is the least active of the three natural estrogens and is one-eightieth the strength of estradiol. It is derived primarily by the conversion of estrone in the liver. Estriol is used in estrogen replacement, especially in triest creams.

Estrogen receptor: is a protein on the cell surface that allows an estrogen molecule to attach and initiate a specific set of commands for the cell to carry out.

Estrone: One of the three forms of natural estrogen produced in women and is one-twelfth the strength of estradiol. Estrone is the most abundant form of circulating estrogen that is present in the postmenopausal woman. Most estrone is in a sulfated form, which prevents it from stimulating breast cells. It is an essential component of triest creams.

Evening primrose oil (EPO): contains the omega-6 essential fatty acid gamma-linolenic acid, or GLA. EPO decreases the formation of inflammatory hormones while promoting those that are anti-inflammatory.

Fibrocystic breast: a common benign condition of the breast. It has been estimated that it occurs on a microscopic level in up to 80 percent of women. Fibrocystic changes are characterized by the abundance of cysts arising from overstimulated breast tissue. Symptoms include breast masses, pain, and a dark green discharge from the nipple.

Fibroid: is a benign tumor of the uterus, which begins as a single smooth muscle but rapidly grows in a swirl-like pattern.

Flavonoids: are plant-derived substances found in fruit, vegetables, grains, bark, roots, stems, flowers, tea, and wine. Flavonoids have many health benefits and are responsible for the attractive colors in plants.

Folic acid: is a B vitamin that plays an important role in the methylation process.

Folinic acid (5-formyl tetrahydrofolate): is an active form of the folate family. Whereas folic acid is synthetic, folinic acid is a natural folate found in foods.

Follicle: is a fluid-filled ovarian cyst that contains an egg. Mature follicles are able to release eggs that can be fertilized.

Follicular phase: see proliferative phase.

Follicular stimulating hormone (FSH): is a hormone that is released by the pituitary gland that stimulates the ovary to produce estrogen and ripens an ovarian follicle. As the ovary ages FSH levels become elevated.

Free radical: is a highly reactive electrically charged substance that can damage molecules in the cell or the cellular matrix.

Full-term gestation: is a pregnancy where the fetus is considered to be mature. The gestational age is greater than thirty-seven weeks.

Gamma-amino-butyric acid (GABA): is a neurotransmitter whose calming and sedative effects prevent an overload of the nervous system. Progesterone and progesterone metabolites, along with allopregnenolone, promote the action of GABA.

Gamma-linoleic acid (GLA): is a derivative of the omega-6 linoleic acid family. GLA promotes the formation of the anti-inflammatory prostaglandin-one series hormones that stop abnormal cell division and decrease platelet adhesion.

Gene: is the basic unit of DNA, which provides the instruction for a cell to make a specific protein.

Genome: the entire collection of genes that is unique to a particular species or an organism.

Gestational diabetes: is a diagnosis made in pregnancy, which is characterized by abnormally high levels of glucose following meals. Insulin resistance secondary to the elevated hormones of pregnancy is the probable cause. Women with gestational diabetes have a greater risk for adult-onset diabetes and breast cancer later in life.

Glucosinolates: are phytonutrients derived from broccoli, cauli-flower, cabbage and Brussels sprouts. Glucosinolates contain both anticancer substances and detoxification boosters.

Gluten: is a protein found in wheat, oats, barley, and rye.

Halogens: are located in Group VII A of the Periodic Table of Ele-ments and are nonmetals. Because halogens have only seven electrons they are considered to be very chemically reactive and generally form salt-like compounds. Included in the halogen family are bromine, chlorine, fluorine, and iodine.

Heavy metals: are metals such as mercury, arsenic, aluminum, lead, nickel, tin, and cadmium that accumulate in the deep tissues of the body. The heavy metals can be removed only by the use of strong chelators. Cadmium is a hormonal disruptor and provides for a low-grade estrogen-like effect on breast cells.

Heart and estrogen/progestin replacement study (HERS): the first large randomized clinical trial involving 2,763 postmenopausal women who were treated with synthetic estrogen and progesterone (Prempro). The average age of participants was 67. Results showed an increased risk of blood clots in the legs and lungs. Prempro did not prevent further heart attacks or death from coronary heart disease in women with a history of heart disease.

Hodgkin's lymphoma (disease): is a cancer of the lymphatic tissue, located in the lymph nodes, spleen, liver, and bone marrow.

Homo sapiens: is the species to which all human beings belong.

Human growth hormone: is a hormone that is released from the pituitary. It regenerates and repairs body tissues while increasing your metabolism. Many have labeled HGH as the true hormone of youth.

Hypertension: is the disorder that is characterized by high blood pressure.

Hypoglycemia: is a condition characterized by low blood sugar, usually less than 70 mg/dl. Symptoms include fatigue, shakiness, and dizziness. Hypoglycemia can be induced by eating carbohydrates, resulting in excessive release of insulin into the bloodstream.

Hypothalmus: is that part of the brain which signals the pituitary gland to release specific hormonal messages. The hypothalamus is composed of nerve cells, and regulates body functions such as temperature, appetite, emotional behavior, and autonomic functions.

Hysterectomy: is the surgical removal of the uterus.

Insulin growth factor hormone type 1 (IGF-1): is made by the liver in direct response to human growth hormone stimulation. IGF-1 encourages cell division and requires careful balancing.

Insulin growth factor binding protein-3 (IGFBP-3): is a protein that binds almost 95 percent of the IGF-1 present in the blood. The rate of IGFBP-3 production is dependent upon human growth hormone levels. IGFBP-3 has demonstrated anti-cancer properties, especially through the promotion of apoptosis of breast cells.

Immune system: is the body's primary defense against foreign invaders and cancer cells.

Indole-3-carbinol (I3C): is derived from the breakdown of glucosinolates found in cruciferous vegetables. I3C, when acted upon by stomach acid, is converted into diindolylmethane (DIMN) and other products such as indolocarbazole.

Indolocarbazole (ICZ): is a by-product of indole-3-carbinol. ICZ has a structure similar to that of the cancer-producing dioxin and increases the production of the carcinogenic 4-hydrox estrogens.

Insulin: is a hormone secreted by the pancreas and controls your blood sugar levels. It also enhances cell division and cancer formation.

Insulin resistance: is a condition in which cells have increasing insensitivities to insulin. The body must then correct this by producing higher levels of insulin.

Interleukin-6 (IL-6): is a molecule which causes inflammatory reactions in the body. Detoxification, estradiol and fish oil decrease their production while fat cells cause an increase. IL-6 is derived from the thymus (TH-1) cells.

Ionic bond: is an electrical attraction between two oppositely charged atoms. One of the atoms is usually metallic and tends to share its electrons with the nonmetallic atom.

Iodine: is an essential element that is in the same chemical family as chlorine. Iodine is very reactive chemically and does not exist as a single atom in nature. The common forms include: 1) two iodine atoms joined together to form molecular I_2 and 2) iodide, which is an iodine atom, combined with either Na (sodium) or K (potassium). Iodine stops abnormal division of breast cells. The thyroid uses iodide in making both T3 and T4.

Irritable bowel syndrome (IBS): is a functional disorder of the bowel, which has both organic and psychological elements. IBS is subdivided into pain, diarrhea, or constipation.

Ketoconazole (Nizoral): is an antifungal pharmaceutical drug, which is thought to act by impairing the formation of the fungal or yeast membrane. An off label use of Nizoral involves the treatment of prostate cancer.

L-glutamine: is the most prevalent amino acid in the bloodstream. The cells that line the intestines use glutamine as their principal source of fuel.

L-tyrosine: is an amino acid that can be converted into dopa and the catechol neurotransmitters (norepinephrine, epinephrine).

Leaky intestine syndrome (leaky gut syndrome): is loss of integrity of the intestinal lining, which causes increased permeability, allowing unwanted molecules or toxins into the bloodstream. These toxins then can activate the immune system, causing unwanted inflammation.

Leptin: is a hormone made by fat cells. It acts at the hypothalamic level of the brain to decrease appetite. Low levels, receptor resistance, and abnormally shaped leptin can result in an increased appetite followed by excessive weight gain.

Letrozole (Femara): is a pharmaceutical drug that lowers estradiol through the inhibition of the enzyme aromatase. Femara is used in the treatment of breast cancer.

Libido: sex drive.

Lignan: is a plant-derived chemical or phytonutrient. It is converted by bacteria living in your intestines into secondary compounds that control estrogen metabolism. Flaxseeds contain lignans that increase the production of the beneficial 2OH estrogen.

Liposome (liposomal): is a spherically shaped bilayer of phospholipids. Various molecules such as EDTA can be encapsulated by the liposome in order to allow enhanced absorption through the intestinal wall.

Lugol's solution: is an iodine/iodide solution developed in the early 1900s. Lugol's solution was used extensively in medical practice to address thyroid diseases. Lugol's solution consists of 10% potassium iodide, 5% iodine, and 85% distilled water.

Luteinizing hormone (LH): is the hormone secreted by the pituitary gland, which triggers the release of an egg from the mature ovarian follicle.

Luteal phase: is the second part of the menstrual cycle, which is characterized by an increase in progesterone production. During the luteal phase of the menstrual cycle the endometrium matures in order to accept and nourish an embryo. The length is generally two weeks.

Lymphatic system: consist of lymphatic vessels, nodes, thymus, and lymphocytes. The lymph system both removes and neutralizes toxins in the body while repelling infectious foreign invaders such as bacteria and viruses.

Magnetic resonance imaging (MRI): A diagnostic test that is performed by a radiologist. A high-power magnet with computer assistance generates images that examine tissues such as the breast.

Melatonin: better known as the sleep hormone, it is produced by a small gland located deep within the brain called the pineal gland. It promotes sleep and is protective of the breast.

Menses (menstrual flow): is the periodic shedding of the endometrium mixed with blood and other debris.

Metabolic syndrome (Syndrome X): is characterized by elevated levels of blood glucose following carbohydrate-laden meals, a decrease in cell sensitivity to insulin, and an increase in circulating insulin in the bloodstream. The inflammatory changes that result from the metabolic syndrome increase the risk of breast cancer and its recurrence.

Metabolic rate: the rate at which energy is released within the body.

Metabolite (downstream): is a breakdown or intermediate product in a biochemical pathway. The metabolite may be more biologically active than the original parent substance.

Metastasis: is the spread of cancer cells from one part of the body to another.

Mitochondria: are the energy factories of the cell. They appear as rod-shaped structures located within the cell and contain only DNA contributed by your mother.

Mitosis: is the process where a cell divides into two genetically identical daughter cells.

Mutagen: is any substance that causes mutations.

Mutate: is to change the molecular structure of DNA.

Neurotransmitter: is a molecule released by a nerve cell in order to send messages to other nerve cells. Two main neurotransmitters include serotonin and catecholamine.

Norepinephrine: is a neurotransmitter in the catecholamine family. L-tyrosine is converted through a series of multiple chemical reactions into norepinephrine.

Nuclear Factor-κB (NF–κB): is a molecule upon being released inside the cell travels to the nucleus where it switches on those genes controlling inflammation. Estradiol prevents excessive activation of NF–κB.

Nucleus: is the sac located inside a cell, which contains the DNA that directs cellular functions.

Oligoantigenic diet: is a selective diet that has a low allergy potential. It may be described as lean and clean. Foods that should be avoided include: wheat (gluten), dairy, soy, corn, alcohol, and processed foods in general. Suggested foods include those that are colorful such as fruits and vegetables.

Oral contraceptives: are birth control pills, which generally contain powerful synthetic estrogens and progestins.

Organic acids: are the downstream metabolites formed during the biologic energy cycle.

Osteoporosis: a condition in which bone mass declines, leading to bone thinning and an increase in bone porosity. Osteoporosis is an inflammatory change most often seen during postmenopause and can increase the chance of bone fracture, especially in the hip and spine.

Oxytocin: is a hormone that is released by the pituitary gland. It causes the smooth muscles of the breast and the pregnant uterus to contract. Oxytocin can also enhance the sensation and lubrication of the vagina.

pH: is a measure of the acidity or alkalinity of a solution. pH has a numerical range from 0 to 14 where 7 is considered to be neutral. The pH of venous blood is said to be optimal at 7.46.

Periodontal inflammation: is a chronic inflammatory process involving the gum and bone surrounding the tooth. This results in bone loss while eventually increasing unwanted tooth mobility.

Pituitary gland: is a pea-size gland at the base of the brain that secretes hormonal messages, which control important glands such as the ovaries, adrenals, thyroid, and testicles.

Phytoestrogens: are compounds found in certain plants and which exhibit weak estrogen-like properties. Soy is a popular phytoestrogen.

Polycystic ovaries (PCOS): is a syndrome that involves abnormal functioning of the ovaries — eggs are not released by the ovary, menstrual cycles are irregular, facial hair increases, and cells are resistant to the effects of insulin.

Prebiotic: describes substances that specific intestinal bacteria require to live. Examples include fiber and oligosaccharides (undigested carbohydrates).

Pregnanes: are metabolites of progesterone formed by the action three enzymes: 5α reductase, 3α-hydroxysteroid oxidoreductase (3α-HSO), and 20α-HSO.

Premarin: is a synthetic conjugated form of estrogen that is derived from the urine of pregnant mares. It contains a number of estrogenic substances, including estrone sulfate, equilenin, dihydroequilin, and equiline. Premarin is at least four times more powerful than estradiol and may remain in the body for several weeks.

Premenstrual syndrome (PMS): is a disorder occurring in the second part of the menstrual cycle. It most often results from a progesterone insufficiency and is characterized by fatigue, bloating, headaches, water retention, moodiness, irritability, anxiety, and depression.

Prempro: is a combination of the synthetic hormones Premarin and Provera. Its use was noted to increase the risk of breast cancer in the WHI study.

Probiotic: are those live microorganisms that when consumed in adequate amounts confer health benefits.

Progesterone: is nature's anti-anxiety or sedating hormone (not to be confused with Provera). Progesterone has been described as a braking system on the effects of estrogen and is important in correcting PMS. Progesterone stops breast cells from dividing and protects against breast cancer. It is produced in large quantities during pregnancy and to a somewhat lesser degree in the luteal phase of the menstrual cycle.

Progestin: is the term applied to include both synthetic and natural progesterone. In the context of this book, progestins refer to the synthetic versions.

Prohormone: a hormone that is essentially inactive unless it is converted by the body into more hormonally active byproducts. Testosterone is a prohormone that is converted into the hormonally active estradiol and dihydrotestosterone. DHEA is converted to testosterone and estradiol.

Proliferative phase: is the phase of the menstrual cycle leading up to ovulation. Estrogen, the primary hormone present during this phase, stimulates the endometrium to grow.

Prostate: is a walnut-sized gland that surrounds the male urethra. The urethra is the tube that carries urine from the bladder to the penis.

Prostate-specific antigen (PSA): is a prognostic marker for benign enlargement of the prostate and prostatic cancer. PSA is measured in the blood and if elevated can be an early warning sign of prostate cancer.

Provera (medroxyprogesterone acetate): is a synthetic progestin that increases unwanted breast cell division and coronary artery spasm. We suggest that you avoid the long-term use of Provera.

Prostaglandins 1, 2, and 3 series (PG1, PG2, PG3): are special types of hormones in the ecosinoid family, which have a very short life but produce very powerful biologic effects. There are three basic types, of which the PG2 are the most inflammation-producing.

Radiation absorbed dose (rad): is a unit of measurement for radiation. A millirad is a thousandth of a rad.

Recommended daily allowance (RDA): is the minimal daily allowance of a specific nutritional component needed by the human body to prevent diseases associated with a deficiency of that component. The RDA for vitamin C is arrived at by the dose needed to prevent scurvy.

Red wine extract (RWE): is a whole food supplement that is made by removing both water and the fleshy part of the red grape while retaining the skin and seeds.

Root canal therapy: is performed after the decay of a tooth has reached its inner pulp and caused irreversible damage. The pulp region of a tooth contains the nerves and blood supply. A dentist will then extract any remaining infected or necrotic pulp and fill the empty canal with a filling.

Self-regulation: The body's ability to maintain an optimum internal environment.

Serotonin: is a neurotransmitter, which is made by the intestine and the brain. It is derived from the amino acid, 5-hydroxytryptophan. Serotonin deficiencies are implicated in depression and cravings for sweets.

Sex hormone binding globulin (SHBG): is a protein that is made by the liver. It controls access to cells by binding up hormones, especially estrogen. Oral administration of hormones can increase the production of SHBG.

Stromal cells (breast): are cells that surround and support the breast cells lining the milk ducts (epithelial cells). Stromal cells are composed of fibroblasts, cells that line the blood vessel (endothelial cells), fat cells (adipocytes), nerve cells, and inflammatory cells (macrophages).

Sulfatase: is an enzyme, which removes the sulfate molecule that is commonly attached to certain hormones such as DHEA and estrone (DHEAS to DHEA, estrone sulfate to estrone). Removing the sulfate allows these hormones to enter the cell and carry out their specific functions. High levels of sulfatase activity are associated with excessive estrogen stimulation of the breast cell with an increase the risk of breast cancer.

Symbiosis: the coexistence or living together of two species that benefit from one another.

Systemic lupus erythematosus (SLE): is an autoimmune disease (self allergy). The body attacks its own tissues, resulting in pain, rashes, and organ destruction.

Tamoxifen: is an anti-cancer drug commonly used to treat estrogen receptor-positive (ER+) breast cancer. Tamoxifen works by competing with estrogen for receptor sites located on the breast cell.

Testosterone: is one of the most potent androgen hormones made in the body. It protects the breast cells from turning cancerous. In women it provides for a sense of well-being, energy, and sex drive. Men benefit by its masculinizing and androgenic effects and have almost forty times the levels seen in women.

Thrombophlebitis: thrombo means *clot* while phlebitis means *inflammation*. Thrombophlebitis is a blood clot in one or more of your veins that results in pain or reddening of the skin. A clot that occurs in the veins deep within the muscle, especially that of the leg, can be life threatening.

Thyroid antibodies: are self-made antibodies that attack the thyroid gland and impair its function. Thyroid peroxidase (TPO) and thyroglobulin antibodies can be detected by blood tests.

Thyroxine (T4): is the main hormone secreted by the thyroid gland and must be enzymatically converted into the active triiodothyronine (T3). Thyroxine contains four iodine atoms, which is why it is referred to as T4.

Thymus: is a gland located in the frontal upper chest area and is involved in T-cell lymphocyte development. It is the primary gland of the lymphatic system.

Tocopherols: are parts of the family of nutrients that make up vitamin E. There are four natural tocopherols: alpha, beta, gamma, and delta. Alpha is the most common form found in supplements, however, other tocopherols, especially gamma, have important health benefits. Studies reported by the media showing vitamin E to have either no effect on or in some cases worsening of diseases are based on those supplements containing only alpha tocopherol and not the preferred combination of the four types listed above.

Transdermal: is a method of hormone replacement that involves application of the hormone to the skin surface for absorption into the blood. It is a popular method for applying estrogen, progesterone, and testosterone. By making use of the skin instead of oral administration, one avoids the inactivation effects of the liver on the hormone.

Triiodothyronine (T3): is the short-acting potent thyroid hormone that controls the energy production of the body. Only 20 percent originates from thyroid gland secretion, while 80 percent is derived from thyroxine (T4). Triiodothyronine contains three iodine atoms.

Tumor Necrosing Factor alpha (TNF-α): is a molecule which is known as an inflammatory cytokine. It leads to tissue inflammation and destruction. Estrogen tends to lower excessive levels.

Visceral adipose tissue (VAT): is the hormonally active inter-abdominal (deep) fat, not to be confused with the fat just below the skin (subcutaneous).

Women's Health Initiative (WHI): randomized controlled trials sponsored by the National Institutes of Health. The effects of the synthetic hormones Prempro and Premarin were evaluated in regard to breast cancer, osteoporosis, heart disease, and strokes.

Xenobiotic: antibiotic elements from outside the human body, which may perform estrogen-like actions.

Xenoestrogens (foreign estrogens): industrial contaminants such as DDT and PCB that possess weak estrogen-like effects. They are endocrine disruptors and are linked to a variety of health issues, including hormonal cancers such as breast.

INDEX

16alpha-hydroxyestrogen, 27-33, 116, 122, 171, 174, 178, 184-185, 216, 246, 263

16alpha-hydroxyestrone, 30, 116, 184, 263

17β-hydroxysteroid dehydrogenase, 17, 19

2-hydroxyestrogen, 18, 23, 27, 29-33, 93, 116, 122, 171, 178, 182, 184-186, 216, 248, 254, 263, 267, 274, 277

2-hydroxyestrone, 116, 184, 267

2-methoxyestrogen, 18-19, 29, 171, 182, 252, 259-260, 262, 274-275

4-hydroxyestrogen, 21, 27, 29-33, 116, 122, 171, 182, 185, 254, 260, 274, 277

4-hydroxyestrone, 116

4-pregnanes, 145

5-hydroxytryptophan, 105-106, 297

5α-pregnanes, 145

A

Acetaminophen, 115

Acne, 150-151, 153, 156, 223

Acromegaly, 169

Adolescence, 13, 37, 46, 245

Adrenal exhaustion, 152, 154

Adrenaline, 72, 98, 278

Aerobic exercise, 59, 100, 234

Allergens, 120

Allopregnenolone, 144, 287

Alpha linolenic acid, 23, 177

Aluminum, 97, 124, 288

Alveoli, 13-14, 197

Amalgams, 111, 278

American Cancer Society, 5, 236

American College of Obstetricians and Gynecologists, 200

American diet, 75, 90, 92-93, 103, 105, 114, 175, 183, 208

American Heart Association, 93

Amino acids, 43, 84, 105, 121

Amylase, 123

Anastrozole, 19, 89, 188, 279

Androgen, 53, 148-149, 155, 259, 262, 279, 298

Andropause, 204-205, 279

Annals of Internal Medicine, 183

Antibiotics, 9, 22, 39, 58, 85, 113-114, 116, 209, 230, 279

Anti-depressants, 50

Anxiety, 1, 46, 52, 104, 123, 143-144, 146-147, 208, 295

Apoptosis, 19, 173, 183, 216, 245, 248, 258, 263, 279, 289

Apple, 80, 82-83, 99, 101, 103, 167, 188, 194, 241, 260, 281

Arimidex, 19, 89, 188, 279

Armour Thyroid, 160

Aromasin, 19, 188

Aromatase, 16-19, 29, 113, 163, 171, 187-188, 216, 231, 248, 250, 252, 266, 268, 272, 279-280, 291

Arsenic, 9, 124, 183, 255, 288

Arthritis, 32, 47, 93-94, 133, 152-153, 178, 203, 220, 284

Aspartame, 98

Asthma, 97, 113

Autocrine, 133

B

Ball ham curls, 62

Ball wall squats, 61

Basal Body Temperature (BBT), 158-160, 280

BCA: See Biocellular analysis (BCA)

Benign prostatic hypertrophy, 205-206

Beta-glucuronidase, 16, 117, 127, 188, 262, 280, 281

Betaine, 123

BIA: See Bioimpedance analysis (BIA)

Bicep band curls, 67

Biest, 138, 215

Bifidobacterium, 112, 121, 123

Biocellular analysis (BCA), 127-128

Bio-identical estrogen, 20, 23, 25, 215

Bioimpedance analysis (BIA), 127-128

Biotin, 180

Birth control pill, 11, 44, 148, 186, 293

Bladder urgency, 15, 214

Bloating, 15, 46, 82, 118, 123, 141, 223, 295

Blood clots, 20, 26, 33-34, 117, 139, 288

Blood pressure, 32, 72, 76, 96, 124, 139, 165-167, 205, 207, 263, 278, 282, 288

Bones, 4, 13, 57, 60, 113-114, 124, 155-156, 172, 177, 187, 229, 280

Boron, 181

Brain, 4, 8, 15, 36, 40-41, 43, 49-51, 57, 80, 82, 90-91, 103-104, 111, 113-114, 116, 128, 144, 151, 155, 157-158, 161-166, 168, 172, 177, 180, 187, 206, 209-210, 221, 229, 278, 280, 282, 288, 290, 292, 294, 297

BRCA1, 10, 98

BRCA2, 10, 98

Breast cancer, 1-11, 14-23, 26-30, 33, 37, 39-40, 43, 55, 69-72, 74-80, 89-93, 97-98, 103, 107-109, 112-118, 122-123, 131, 135, 139-140, 145, 147, 149, 152, 155, 159, 162-163, 165, 167, 170-176, 178-179, 182, 184-191, 194-201, 203, 205, 209-214, 216-217, 220, 230-232, 245, 247-280, 282, 284, 287, 291-292, 295, 297, 299

Breast Care Supplement Program, 3, 172

Breast Massage, 2, 69-70

Breast self-exam (BSE), 191-193, 201, 236

Breast surveillance triad, 191, 195, 197

Breast tenderness, 15, 28, 41, 46, 70, 141, 160-161, 192

Breast-feeding, 11, 38, 69, 76

BreastSecure, 3, 172, 184-186, 188, 206, 234, 243, 280

Bromine, 176, 287

BSE: See Breast self-exam (BSE)

Buffalo hump, 164

C

Cadmium, 9, 38, 117, 124, 257-258, 288

Caffeine, 78, 97-98, 174, 235, 262

Calcium, 96, 105, 123, 171-172, 180, 184-185, 188, 197, 206-207, 234, 257, 281

Calcium D-glucarate, 123, 171-172, 184-185, 188, 206, 234, 280-281

Canadian Journal of Surgery, 174, 255

Canadian National Breast Screening Study No. 1, 200

Candida, 81-82, 85, 89, 116, 123, 147, 281

Carbohydrate, 50, 79-80, 82, 85, 88, 90, 95, 102-103, 114, 118, 121, 165, 168, 226, 235, 247, 282, 288, 292, 294

Carotene, 78, 281

Catechol-O-methyltransferase (COMT), 182, 252, 255, 261, 266, 271, 274

CDSA: See Complete digestive stool analysis (CDSA)

Celexa, 104

Celiac disease, 128

Cell matrix, 6-8, 108, 110, 113, 210-211, 216

Cellular matrix, 8, 109, 210, 213, 281, 286

Chelation Therapy, 107, 124-126, 129, 207, 211, 214, 224, 236, 247, 251, 282

Chemotherapy, 3, 29, 123, 163, 196, 210-211, 262

Chinese medicine, 126, 127, 211

Chlorine, 100, 176, 287, 290

Cholesterol, 116-117, 137, 143, 151-152, 167, 169, 181, 187, 205, 207, 229, 282

Chromium, 181

Cigarette smoke, 115, 124

Cimetidine, 115

Circadian rhythms, 80

Cleanse, Add, Nourish program, 2, 107, 120, 122-123, 129, 213, 281

Climara, 139

Clitoris, 150-151

Colonic therapy, 126

Colonocytes, 113, 281

Committee on Biological Effects of Ionizing Radiation, 198

Complete digestive stool analysis (CDSA), 127

COMT: See Catechol-O-methyltransferase (COMT)

Copper, 86, 181, 187

CoQ-10, 189

corpus luteum, 41, 43, 45

Cortisol, 36, 42, 72, 98, 104, 134, 136, 144, 148, 152, 155, 164-166, 251, 267, 274, 277-278, 282

Coumestrol, 21, 23

C-reactive protein, 127, 251

CYP450, 114, 116, 252

Cytokines, 115, 283

Cytomel, 160

D

Daidzein, 22

Dairy, 87, 228, 240

Dehydroepiandrosterone (DHEA), 16, 18-19, 36, 54, 98, 136, 148, 152-156, 161, 205-206, 208, 214, 249, 259, 278-279, 282-283, 295, 297

Dementia, 32, 126, 132, 152, 155, 165, 187, 214

Deoxyribonucleic acid (DNA), 1, 6, 7, 8, 9, 27, 30, 31, 98, 107, 110, 113, 179, 181, 182, 210, 216, 249, 265, 266, 268, 277, 279, 283, 284, 287, 292, 293

Depression, 15, 43-44, 46, 49, 52, 54, 74, 93-94, 97, 104, 141, 144, 147, 159, 162, 203-205, 214, 220, 223, 279, 295, 297

Detox Questionnaire, 123

Detoxification, 8-10, 16, 24-25, 33, 43-45, 58, 82, 107-108, 110, 114-115, 117-118, 120, 122-124, 126-129, 133, 149, 158, 162, 188, 205, 207-208, 210-213, 216, 220, 223-225, 229, 233, 236, 282-283, 287, 289

DHA: See Docosahexaenoic acid (DHA)

DHEA: See Dehydroepiandrosterone (DHEA)

DHT: See Dihydrotestosterone (DHT)

Diabetes, 83, 90, 111, 133, 155, 166-167, 203, 207, 211, 220, 246, 287

Dihomo-gamma-linolenic acid, 92

Dihydroequilin, 28, 294

Dihydrotestosterone (DHT), 149, 283, 295

Diindolylmethane (DIMN), 123, 171-172, 184-186, 249, 277, 280, 282, 284, 289

Dimercapto propane sulfonic acid (DMPS), 125, 282

Dimercapto succinic acid (DMSA), 125, 282

DIMN: See Diindolylmethane (DIMN)

Dioxin, 21, 235, 272-273, 289

Diuretic, 99, 143

DMPS: See Dimercapto propane sulfonic acid (DMPS)

DMSA: See Dimercapto succinic acid (DMSA)

DNA: See Deoxyribonucleic acid (DNA)

Docosahexaenoic acid (DHA), 23, 93, 95, 177-178, 234, 249

Dr. Jekyll and Mr. Hyde, 92

E

EBCT: See Electron-beam computed tomography (EBCT)

Eczema, 113, 128, 223, 284

EDTA: See Ethylene diamine tetraacetic acid (EDTA)

Eicosanoids, 90, 272

Eicosapentaenoic acid (EPA), 23, 93, 95, 177, 178, 234

Electron-beam computed tomography (EBCT), 207

Endocrine, 36, 43, 46, 110, 133, 152, 169, 221, 247, 257, 259, 261, 264-265, 268-270, 299

Endogenous toxins, 107

Endometriosis, 15, 28, 44, 143, 174, 187, 256, 284

Enzymes, 16, 19, 28, 39, 85, 89, 95-96, 111, 113-116, 121, 123-124, 129, 157-158, 182, 231, 256, 262, 264, 277, 282-283, 294

EPA: See Eicosapentaenoic acid (EPA)

Equilin, 28, 274

Equol, 22

ER– cells, 27, 29

ER+ cells, 27, 29, 178, 184-185, 188, 297

Estradiol, 15-19, 21, 28-29, 31, 36, 116-117, 135, 137-140, 161, 171, 185, 187, 206, 214-215, 230, 246, 249, 251-252, 254, 259-260, 262-263, 265-267, 269-271, 274-275, 277-280, 282, 284-285, 289, 291, 293-295

Estriol, 15-16, 21, 28, 30, 116, 137-138, 140, 215, 259-260, 262, 267, 271, 285

Estrogen, 2, 6, 10, 13-16, 18, 21-23, 25-33, 36, 41, 44-53, 55, 58, 70, 92, 107, 110, 113-114, 116-117, 122, 124, 132, 135-138, 140-148, 152, 155-156, 160-161, 163, 171-172, 174, 178, 184-188, 192, 196-197, 203-206, 208, 211, 213-216, 230-231, 246-248, 250-256, 258, 260-265, 267-272, 274-275, 277-286, 288, 291, 294-295, 297, 299

Estrogen deficiency, 15, 49, 132, 135, 278

Estrogen dominance, 14, 44-47, 49, 143, 146

Estrone, 15-16, 18-19, 28, 116-117, 137-140, 215, 250, 259, 265, 271, 277-278, 282, 285, 294, 297

Ethylene diamine tetraacetic acid (EDTA), 125, 126, 207, 236, 243, 247, 251, 282, 284, 291

F

Facial hair, 150-151, 294

Far-infrared sauna, 126

Fat-burning zone, 59-60

Fatigue, 2, 15, 43, 46, 48-49, 53-54, 61, 79, 107, 113, 123, 128, 136, 151, 153-154, 157-159, 165, 204, 208, 279, 288, 295

Fats, 78-79, 82, 87, 90-95, 102, 114, 118, 121, 165, 282

FDA: See Food and Drug Administration (FDA)

FEM Centre Breast Care Pyramid, 19, 24, 37, 55, 57-59, 140, 212, 280

Femara, 19, 89, 188, 280, 291

Fiber, 9, 22, 78-82, 84, 88-89, 121, 135, 226, 281, 294

Fibrocystic breast disease, 14, 174, 262

Fibroid, 15, 28, 30, 36, 44, 47, 87, 139, 141, 143, 160, 187, 286

Fibromyalgia, 220

Fish, 3, 38-39, 86, 89, 93, 95, 124, 172-173, 177-178, 206, 227, 233-234, 243, 249, 267, 289

Fish oil, 38, 95, 172, 177-178, 206, 234, 243, 249, 289

Flaxseed, 23, 93-95, 177, 227, 248, 256, 291

Flour, 84, 95, 226, 235

Fluorine, 100, 176, 287

Folic acid, 38, 76, 105, 171, 180, 182-183, 232, 245, 254, 271, 280, 286

Follicular phase, 47, 286

Follicular Stimulating Hormone (FSH), 36, 41, 49, 51, 286

Food Additives and Coloring Agents, 97

Food and Drug Administration (FDA), 178, 194, 215

Food sensitivity testing, 127-128

Free radicals, 7, 103, 107, 162, 179, 279

Fruits, 8, 76, 78, 80, 82-83, 89, 182, 226, 229, 241, 281, 293

FSH: See Follicular Stimulating Hormone (FSH)

Functional hypothyroidism, 158

Fungi, 89, 120, 279, 281

Fuzzy memory, 2, 15, 46, 113, 132, 141, 152, 154, 159, 204

G

GABA: See Gamma-aminobutyric acid (GABA)

Gallbladder disease, 118, 223

Gamma-aminobutyric acid (GABA), 151, 287

Gamma-linolenic acid, 92, 285

Gel/Cream Application, 141

Genistein, 22

Gestational diabetes, 43, 287

Glucosinolate, 78, 287, 289

Glycemic Index, 4, 82-83, 226, 239

Grain, 8, 76, 83, 89, 182, 215, 226, 269, 286

Gut-associated lymphatic tissue, 115

H

H. pylori, 112, 122

Halogen, 176, 287

Headaches, 2, 46, 49, 52, 74, 97, 128, 159, 223, 295

Heart, 2, 4-5, 8, 15, 20, 26, 29, 32-33, 51, 54, 57, 59-60, 78, 83, 90-93, 96, 102-103, 111-116, 125-127, 133, 139, 142-144, 147, 151, 155, 159, 162-163, 166-169, 172, 177-178, 183, 186-187, 203-207, 211, 214, 219, 221, 229-232, 237, 280, 282-283, 288, 299

Heart disease, 2, 5, 8, 15, 20, 26, 32-33, 78, 83, 90, 93, 111, 125-127, 133, 139, 142-143, 147, 155, 162-163, 167, 178, 183, 186, 203-205, 207, 211, 214, 219, 231-232, 237, 288, 299

Heartburn, 74, 112, 118, 223

Heavy menstrual flows, 15, 143

Heavy metals, 7, 38-39, 58, 108, 111, 113, 115, 117, 124-125, 178, 183, 211, 235, 237, 250, 282, 288

HGH: See Human growth hormone (HGH)

High-sensitivity C-reactive protein, 118, 127, 182

Hippocampus, 165

Homeopathy, 126

Hormone replacement therapy (HRT), 1, 2, 4, 20, 25, 28, 33, 137, 149, 160, 252-253, 258, 260, 263-264, 266, 274

Hot flashes, 2, 15, 47-52, 123, 132, 141, 154, 160, 214-215

HRT: See Hormone replacement therapy (HRT)

Human growth hormone (HGH), 13, 50, 54, 135-136, 139-140, 148, 154, 168-169, 205-206, 229, 288-289

Hunter-gatherers, 76, 259

Hydrochloric acid, 85, 121

Hyperthyroidism, 157-159

Hypoglycemia, 112, 166-167, 288

I

IGF-1: See Insulin-like Growth Factor 1 (IGF-1)

in utero, 39

in vitro, 179, 257

in vivo, 179, 249, 258, 265-266, 268

Indole-3-carbinol, 185-186, 249, 284, 289

Initiation, 5-7, 10, 141, 171, 245, 249

Insecticides, 39

Insomnia, 15, 46-47, 54, 107, 123, 163, 204, 214

Insulin, 13, 32, 42-43, 50, 72, 80, 93, 112, 118, 135-136, 141, 147, 155, 166-168, 213, 232, 255-256, 265, 270, 274, 287-289, 292, 294

Insulin-like Growth Factor 1 (IGF-1), 168, 169, 170, 289

IntestRestore, 206-207, 213, 225-226, 228-229, 233-234, 243

Inuits, 93

Iodide, 157, 174, 176, 253, 269, 290-291

Iodine-loading test, 175-176

Irritable bowel syndrome, 118, 122, 220, 223, 290

Isoflavones, 21-23

J

Janus effect, 18, 26

Journal of the American Medical Association, 114, 245, 250, 253, 263, 267, 271, 274

Journal of the National Cancer Institute, 18, 252, 257, 267, 269, 274

K

Ketoconazole, 89, 290

Kidney, 29, 96, 99, 109, 116, 142, 157, 169, 181, 219, 239, 278, 283

Kupffer cells, 115

L

Lactiferous duct, 13-14

Lactobacillus, 112, 123

Lead, 18, 21, 28, 30, 38-39, 43, 47-49, 51, 53, 72, 79, 93, 98, 113, 116-118, 124, 144, 147, 150, 156, 158, 162, 165-167, 204-205, 210, 214, 263, 267, 280-282, 285, 288

Leaky gut syndrome, 112-113, 115, 117, 120, 290

Legumes, 21, 78, 88-89, 226, 233, 239

Leptin, 50, 290

Letrozole, 19, 89, 188, 280, 291

Levothyroid, 160

Lexapro, 104

LH: See Luteinizing hormone (LH)

Lignans, 21, 23, 291

Linoleic acid, 92, 284, 287

Lipase, 85, 95, 123

Lipopolysaccharides, 116

Liver-intestinal detoxification system, 43, 45-46, 114, 118, 123, 229

L-tyrosine, 105-106, 290, 293

Luteal phase, 41, 50, 291, 295

Luteinizing hormone (LH), 41, 291

Lycopene, 206

Lymphatic breast massage, 69

M

M. D. Anderson Cancer Center, 188

Macular degeneration, 126

Magnesium, 95, 180-181

Male pattern baldness, 150

Male wellness, 203

Mammary lobe, 13-14

Mammogram, 174, 191, 194-201, 236, 284

Manganese, 181

MDR: See Minimum Daily Requirement (MDR)

Melatonin, 50, 54, 80, 134, 136, 154, 161-163, 168, 205-206, 250, 292

Menopausal zest, 54

Menopause, 11, 14-16, 25, 32-33, 36-37, 43-45, 49-53, 131, 141, 143, 148, 160, 204-205, 220, 251, 264, 273, 279

Menstrual cycle, 40-42, 47, 135, 147, 159, 199, 291, 294-295

Mercury, 9, 38-39, 86, 111, 124, 178, 227-278, 288

Metastasis, 145, 166-167, 210, 231, 292

Methylation, 29, 182, 232, 261, 265, 286

Methylenetetrahydrofolate reductase (MTHFR), 182, 245, 248, 254-255

Mineral, 46, 80, 88, 95-96, 100, 105, 111, 121, 123, 128, 173, 178-180, 211, 226, 228

Minimum Daily Requirement (MDR), 178

Mitosis, 13, 27, 41, 292

Molybdenum, 181

Monosaturated fats, 91, 94

Monosodium glutamate (MSG), 97-98

Mood swings, 2, 46, 48, 79, 132, 208, 223

MSG: See Monosodium glutamate (MSG)

MTHFR: See Methylenetetrahydro-folate reductase (MTHFR)

Multivitamin, 3, 80, 171-172, 178-179, 181, 234

N

N-acetylcysteine (NAC), 115, 230

National Health and Nutrition Survey, 175

Nature-Thyroid, 160

NeuroResearch, 105, 243, 257

Niacin, 180

Night sweats, 15, 47, 49-52, 54, 132, 141, 143, 161, 208, 214-215

Nitrite, 97

Non-identical hormone, 20

Norepinephrine, 104-105, 290, 293

Nutrition, 38, 58-59, 74, 77, 79-80, 89, 104, 206, 210-211, 213, 233, 245-248, 250, 254, 256-259, 265, 268-269, 270

Nuts and seeds, 95, 227

O

Oils, 78, 87, 90, 92, 94-96, 123, 227, 235

Oligoantigenic diet, 120, 293

Omega-3 fatty acids, 3, 23, 38, 86, 91-95, 172-173, 177-178, 206, 234, 268

Omega-6 fatty acids, 91-94, 178, 268, 284-285, 287

Oral contraceptives, 11, 293

Organic acid/dysbiosis analysis, 127-128

Osteoporosis, 15, 32, 60, 97, 142-143, 156, 169, 203, 214, 293, 294, 299

Ovarian cancer, 10, 255, 261, 270

Ovaries, 15-16, 36, 40-41, 43, 45-47, 49, 51-53, 90, 133, 142, 144, 148, 151, 160, 186, 212, 285, 294

Overstimulation, 15, 19, 21, 28, 113, 117, 145, 198, 230, 281

Ovulation, 36, 38, 40-41, 45, 48, 50, 52, 142, 144, 192, 295

P

Pancreatin, 85

Pantothenic acid, 180, 232

Paracrine, 133

Parasites, 113, 116, 120, 123

Paxil, 104

Pectoral Squeeze, 70-71

Perimenopause, 28, 36, 45, 48-52, 54-55, 208

Pesticides, 7-8, 39, 58, 76, 100, 108, 113-114, 121, 176, 235, 257

PG1: See Prostaglandin 1 (PG1)

Phase One of Perimenopause, 49-51

Phase Two of Perimenopause (Early Menopause), 50-52

Phytochemical, 78, 252

Phytoestrogen, 20-23, 266, 273, 294

Plastics, 9, 39, 58, 114

PMS: See Premenstrual syndrome (PMS)

Polycystic ovaries, 43, 294

Polycystic ovary syndrome, 167, 246

Polyunsaturated fats, 91-92, 261

Postmenopause, 2, 15, 22, 32, 36-37, 45, 52-55, 146, 148, 197, 220, 285, 293

Potassium, 176, 181, 278, 290-291

Poultry, 85-86, 89, 160, 228, 233

Prednisone, 164

Pregnancy, 11, 16, 29, 37-38, 41, 43-44, 47, 76, 142-143, 147, 163, 186, 216, 271-272, 284, 286-287, 295

Pregnenolone, 54, 136, 151-154, 205-206, 214, 282

Premarin, 18, 20, 25-26, 28, 30, 33, 294-295, 299

Premenopause, 14, 37, 43-49, 55, 220, 285

Premenstrual syndrome (PMS), 41, 43, 44, 46, 55, 141, 146, 295

Prempro, 20, 25-26, 33, 75, 122, 288, 295, 299

Procyanidins, 187

Progesterone, 13-14, 18-19, 25, 36, 41, 43, 45, 47-48, 50, 52, 70, 136, 142-147, 151-152, 161, 192, 197, 206, 246, 249, 253-254, 260, 262, 264-265, 269, 271, 273, 278, 282, 284, 287-288, 291, 294-295, 299

Progestin, 25-26, 144, 261, 288, 295-296

Prohormone, 149, 155, 283, 295

Prolactin, 13

Propagation, 5-6, 10, 27

Prostaglandin 1 (PG1), 92, 296

Prostate cancer, 17, 182, 203-205, 249, 258-259, 270, 290, 296

Prostate-specific antigen (PSA), 207, 296

Protein, 6, 22-23, 78-80, 82, 84-86, 88-89, 95, 102, 104, 106, 114, 117-118, 121, 135, 164-165, 168, 170, 226-227, 229, 233, 247, 264, 268, 281-282, 285, 287, 289, 297

Proteinase, 123

Provera, 25-26, 144, 295, 296

Prozac, 104

Psoriasis, 113, 223

R

Radiation, 8-9, 108, 123, 163, 194, 196, 198, 210, 296

Recommended Daily Allowance (RDA), 173, 179, 296

Red meat, 87, 105, 233

Red wine extract, 19, 123, 171-172, 184-185, 187-188, 206, 234, 280, 296

REM sleep, 162

Reproductive Compartments, 2, 35, 45, 47, 52

Reproductive phase, 36, 39, 43-44

Resistance training, 60-61, 169, 234

Resveratrol, 21, 23, 187, 206, 246, 248, 258, 265, 270, 275

Root canals, 111

S

Saliva, 16, 128, 134, 140, 163, 260

Salt, 78, 96, 175, 226, 272, 277, 281, 287

Saturated fat, 8, 85-86, 91, 235

Saw palmetto, 206

Seated tricep extension, 66

Second Brain, 2, 111

Selenium, 115, 181, 183, 206, 248, 250, 255, 283

Serotonin, 15, 50, 80, 104-105, 293, 297

Sex hormone binding globulin (SHBG), 135, 297

Shocked ovaries, 47

Silymarin, 115, 231

Sitting latissimus row, 65

Sleeping pills, 50

Slow acetylators, 115

Sodium benzoate, 97-98

Soy, 21-23, 85, 88, 92, 102, 226, 233, 240, 248, 278-280, 293-294

Splenda, 101

Standing lateral raises, 68

Stationary lunges, 63

Stomach ulcers, 112

Strawberry Almond Super Protein Shake, 229

Stress reduction, 23, 58-59, 71, 104, 206, 213, 216, 234

Stroke, 1-2, 26, 33-34, 78, 111, 117, 139, 299

Sugar, 79-80, 84-85, 89, 103, 164, 166-167, 213, 235, 239, 241, 281, 288-289

Sulfation, 18, 230

Synthetic estrogen, 20-21, 26, 28, 30, 149, 160, 197, 288, 293

Synthroid, 157, 160

T

Tamoxifen, 123, 189, 267, 297

Taoist Breast Massage, 69

TBG: See Thyroid binding globulin (TBG)

Testicular cancer, 206

Testosterone, 18-19, 36, 52-54, 136, 141-142, 147-151, 155-156, 161, 204-205, 208, 214, 248, 252, 262, 268-269, 279-280, 282-283, 295, 298-299

Thermograms, 11, 145, 191, 199, 201, 236

Thermography, 11, 145, 191, 194-196, 199-201, 236, 243, 255, 263

Thiamine, 180

Thyroid binding globulin (TBG), 135

Thyroid hormone, 13, 54, 135, 139, 156-159, 165, 177, 205-206, 250, 283, 299

Thyroid stimulating hormone (TSH), 157-158

Thyrolar, 160

Thyroxine, 36, 157-158, 160, 177, 253, 290, 298-299

Toxemia, 114

Toxic load, 108, 110-111, 127, 158

Toxins, 7, 9, 38, 44, 58, 69, 89, 99, 104, 107-109, 111-114, 117, 120-121, 126-127, 129, 158, 213, 225, 230, 281-283, 290-291

Traditional medicine, 7, 28, 58, 74, 107, 113, 134-135, 158, 179, 196, 199, 203, 207, 210

Trans-fats, 91

Triest, 138-140, 161, 215, 285

Triglycerides, 117, 139

Triiodothyronine, 36, 135-136, 157-158, 160, 177, 253, 283, 290, 298-299

Troches, 139-140, 145

Tryptophan, 80

TSH: See Thyroid stimulating hormone (TSH)

Twenty-Minute Eating Rule, 106, 233

U

University of Alabama, 183

Urine provocation test, 125

Uterus, 13, 25, 36, 142-147, 160, 186, 258, 268, 284, 286, 289, 293

V

Vaccinations, 39

Vaginal dryness, 49, 51, 54, 141, 214

Vaginal sonography, 143

Vegetables, 9, 21, 76, 78, 80-81, 85, 89, 93, 182-183, 185, 226, 233, 239, 281, 286, 289, 293

Vioxx, 32

Viruses, 120, 291

Visceral adipose tissue, 103, 299

Vitamin, 9-10, 19, 44, 46, 58, 70, 76, 78, 80, 88, 95-96, 105, 111, 121-122, 125, 174, 178-182, 207, 211, 216, 226, 231-232, 258, 273-274, 279, 281, 286, 296, 298

Vitamin A, 78, 180, 281

Vitamin B12, 76, 180, 182, 274

Vitamin B2, 180

Vitamin B6, 44, 180, 182, 274

Vitamin C, 122, 125, 179-180, 211, 279, 296

Vitamin D, 10, 19, 180-181, 216, 258, 273

Vitamin D3, 180-181, 273

Vitamin E, 70, 174, 179-180, 207, 279, 298

Vivelle, 139

W

Waist-to-hip ratio, 103

Walking, 59, 60, 234

Water, 9, 18, 21, 44, 58, 76, 78, 93, 96, 99-101, 106, 111, 117, 123, 124, 128, 141, 143, 177, 186, 223, 225, 228, 233, 235, 240, 281, 291, 295-296

Weight gain, 2, 43, 46, 49, 50, 53, 54, 59, 83, 104, 107, 123, 132, 136, 141, 142, 147, 156, 159, 160, 204, 208, 223, 232, 283, 290

Wellbutrin, 104

WHI: See Women's Health Initiative Study (WHI)

Window of Opportunity, 32, 33

Women's Health Initiative Study (WHI), 25-26, 28, 30-33, 117, 131, 137, 140, 295, 299

X

Xenobiotics, 39

Xenoestrogens, 20-21, 23, 38-39, 76, 117, 245, 270, 299

X-ray, 194, 197, 210

Xylitol, 101

Z

Zinc, 95, 122, 180-181, 206

Zoloft, 104